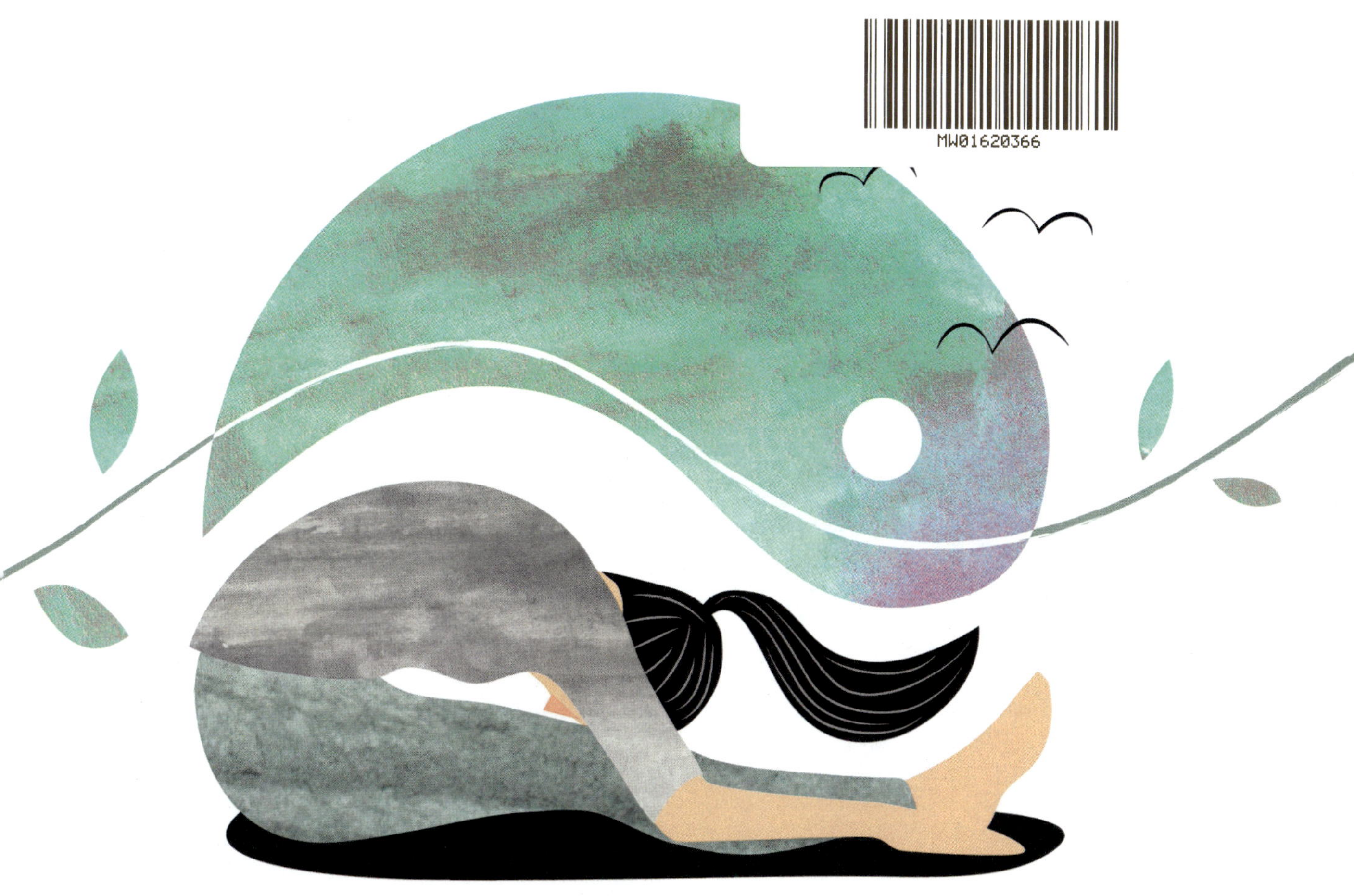

Welcome

Why is self-care such a challenge? Knowing how important it is to take care of ourselves, why do we struggle so often to find the time or the energy to do it? Sometimes even to be kind to ourselves?

Chances are, when you think of self-care, you picture any number of hobbies or activities you'd love to fit into your day if only you had the time: massages, pedicures, a swim, a sunrise meditation. Social media is awash with smoothies, mantras, and wellness rituals that are guaranteed to revolutionize your life. But while these pursuits are undoubtedly positive and beneficial, they're only a part of your self-care story.

The real challenge of self-care comes with learning to listen to yourself so that you can figure out your needs and address them. Feeling frazzled after a difficult day? Perhaps ten minutes standing in the back yard with a warm drink would give you the chance to reset. Struggling to get going after a particularly bad night's sleep? Maybe take a few moments to sit quietly and focus on your breath.

Finding a balance of different self-care rituals that fit with the way you feel and what your body is telling you means giving yourself permission to do whatever you need to at that moment, without feeling selfish. Whether that's letting off steam, taking a little time to be alone, exercising, or enjoying a piece of chocolate cake—it's about what's happening inside of you. Your well-being and wellness come first. It's time to make time for yourself.

---

www.breathemagazine.co.uk

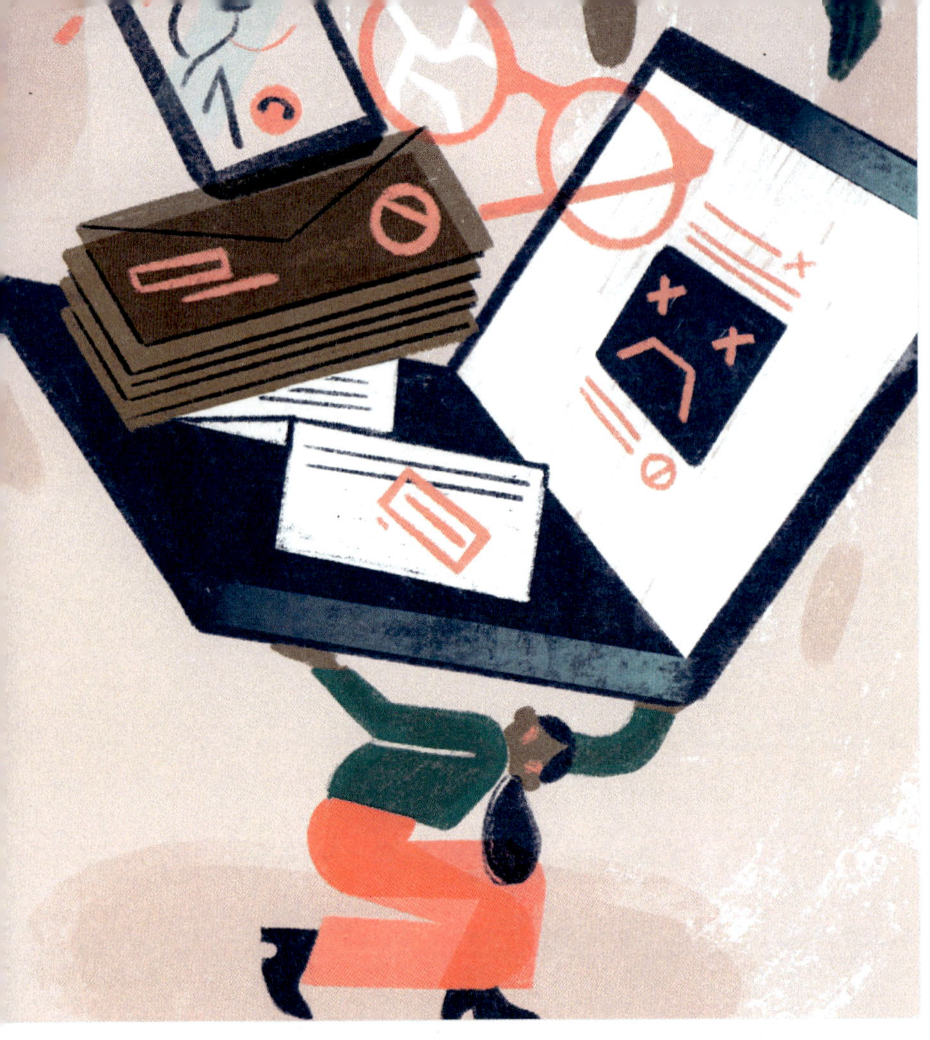

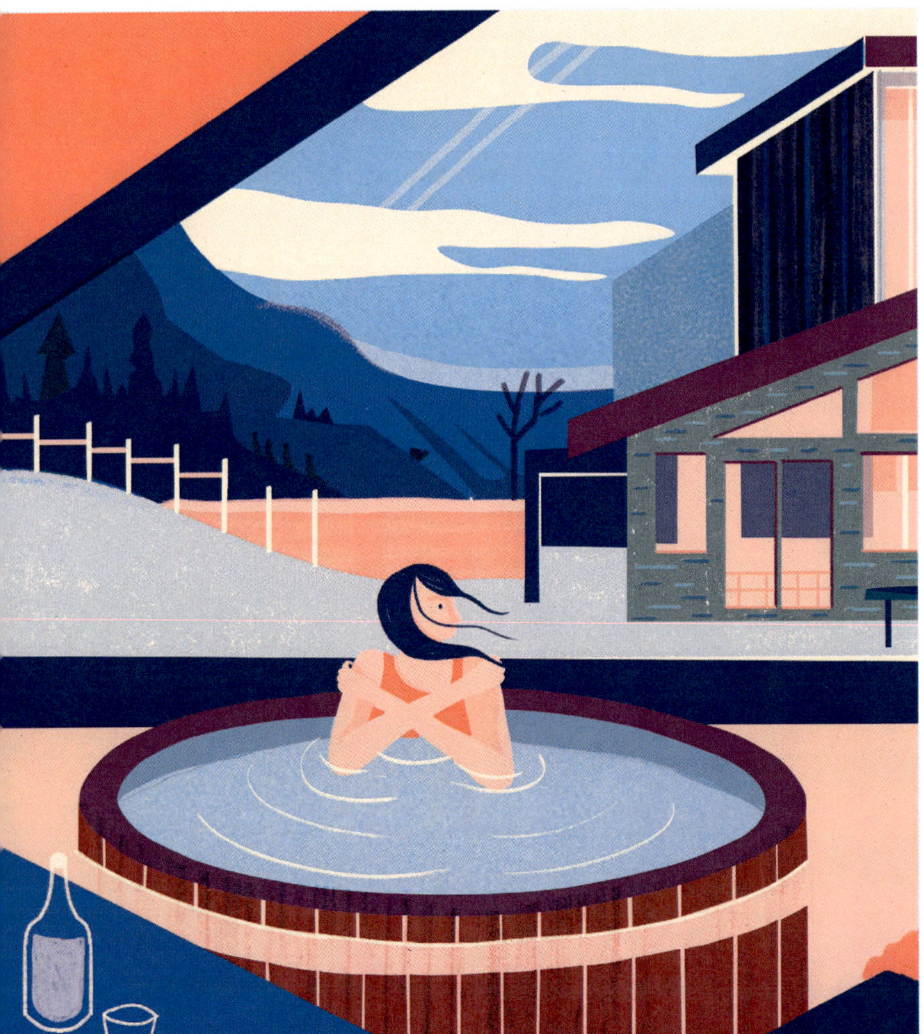

Contents

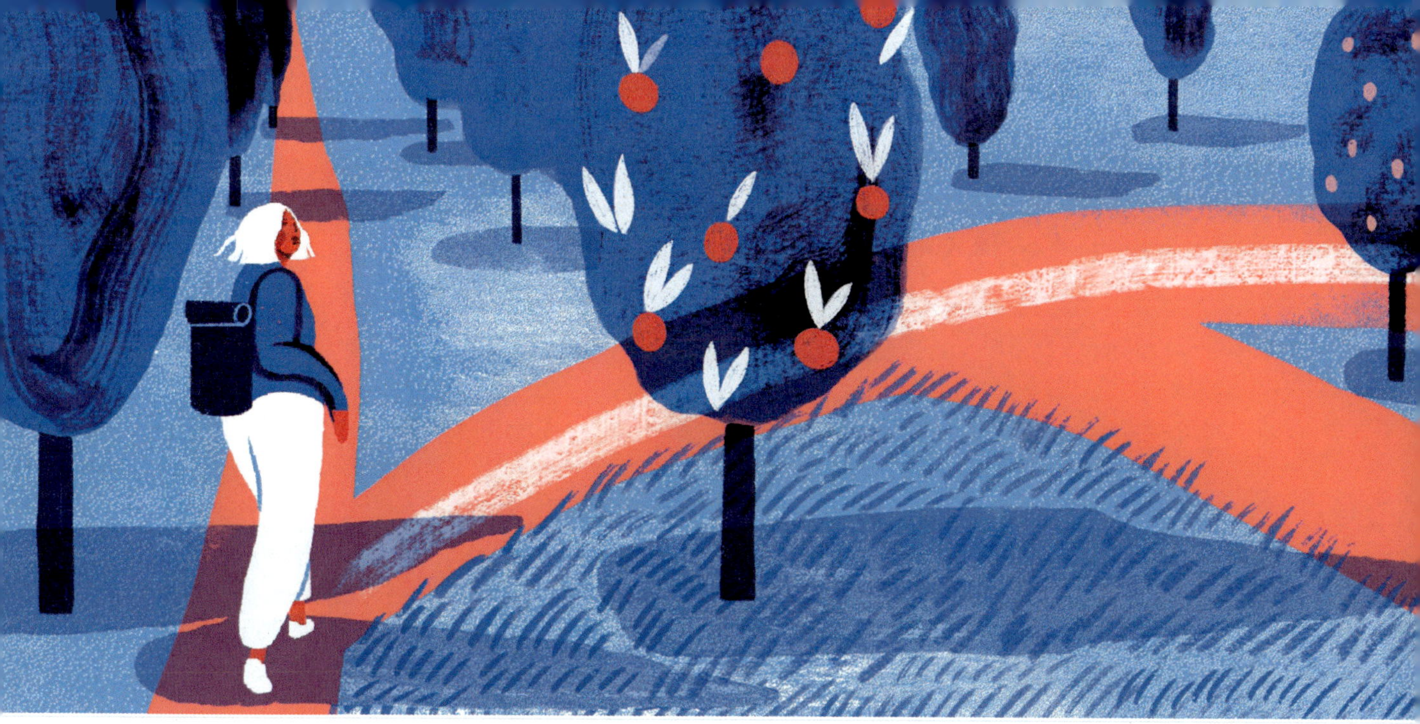

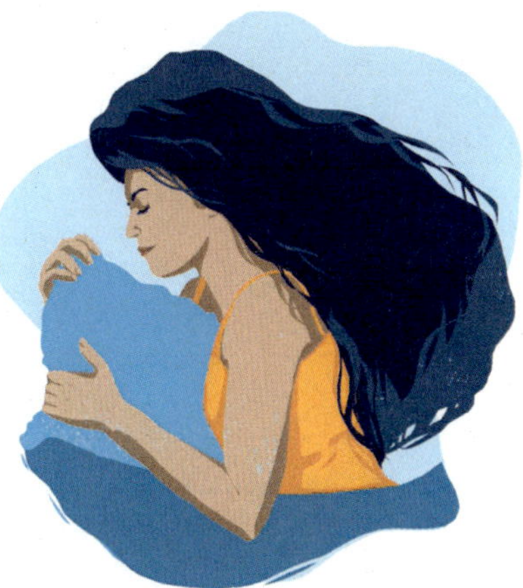

Design: Jo Chapman. **Editorial**: Susie Duff, Catherine Kielthy, Jane Roe. **Publisher**: Jonathan Grogan. **Cover illustration**: Carla Llanos.
Produced by Guild of Master Craftsman Publications Ltd. 86 High Street, Lewes, BN7 1XN, United Kingdom.

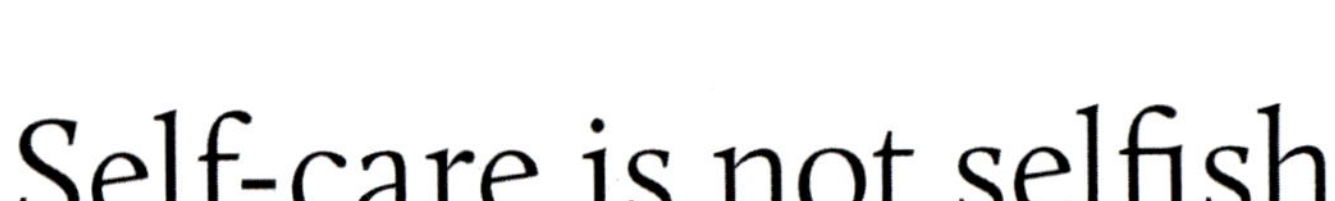

Self-care is not selfish

A trend, a buzzword, a passing fad—self-care has been called many things, but increasingly these days it's a tool for self-preservation. Against the backdrop of a global pandemic, the threat of which is both physical and mental, the need to pay careful attention to body, mind, and soul is perhaps more important than ever

The history and origins of self-care are surprisingly complex. Used as a political weapon against immigrants, reclaimed by minority groups, and with roots in care for the mentally ill, it's a term that's been defined and redefined time and again.

The new radical

Today's more homogenized, Western view of self-care began with the ancient Greeks. According to Rhode Island University scholar Stephanie M. Batters: "For Foucault and the ancient Greeks, it was counterproductive not to focus on the self, and a keen self-awareness was vital for participation in social and political life. Care of the self, then, became a focal point for individual freedom, positive relationships with others, and, potentially, ethical participation in politics."

In the 1960s revolutionary American writer and feminist Audre Lorde breathed new life into this idea with her book, *A Burst of Light*. Written as she battled cancer for the second time, Audre referred to self-care as a political act: "Caring for myself is not self-indulgence," she wrote. "It is self-preservation, and that is an act of political warfare."

In the last decade, self-care might still be regarded as a political act (albeit through a softer filter). In a world that celebrates self-sacrifice, taking care of your own needs first has become a radical decision. Not because you're selfish or, worse, narcissistic, but because you recognize that your household, your work team, you yourself, are not going to survive otherwise.

What gift can you give yourself?

Jo is a 41-year-old single mom to two teenagers. The new normal has been tough on her. Her nearly-but-not-quite adults require her to be emotionally strong and she must still provide for them, but with less adult contact and outside support it's a daily struggle.

Recognizing that her feelings were beginning to act against her well-being, she looked for a way to provide a boost to her day, a mental injection of positivity. She created her own self-care box. Radical? Perhaps not, but this act is practical, positive, and proactive. She said: "I have to be my own advocate. My mental health has to come first otherwise I cannot be there for my children. They're anxious and worried about the future of course, we all are, but if all I want to do is hide away and shut out the world, I can't do anything to help them."

Jo's box is a simple but effective gift to herself. Her favorite chocolate, a book, candles, some reminders of great vacations and times with her children. A few notes written to herself reminding her of her own self-worth become renegade acts of self-care that will see her through turbulent times.

Not everyone's experience of the pandemic has been like Jo's. Some have found themselves completely alone, others surrounded. Acts of self-care will differ for every family, couple, or single setup. It's often seen as a deeply feminine term, something men might struggle to access or apply to themselves. A concept that perhaps has run its course as wider society accepts the vital importance of robust mental health.

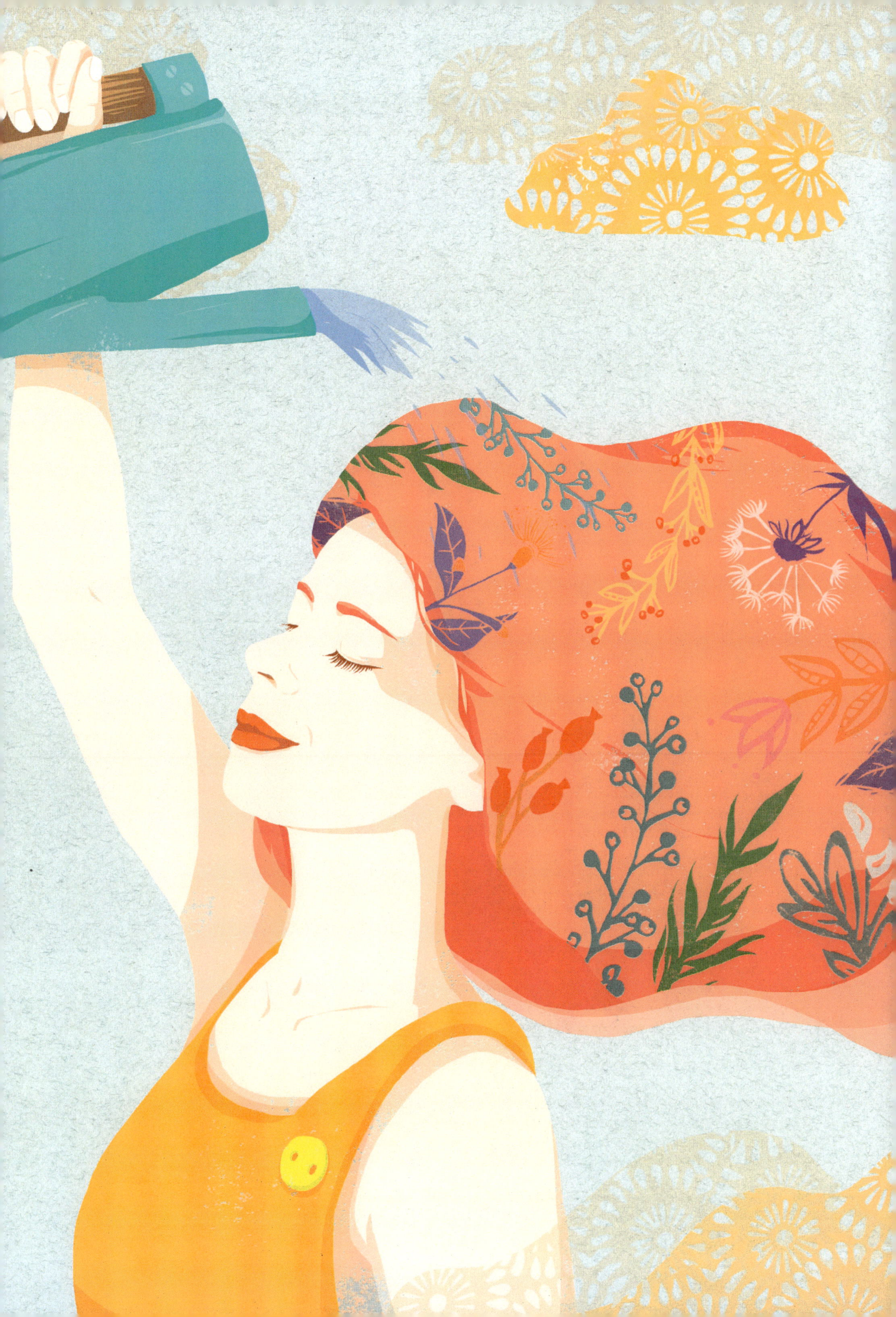

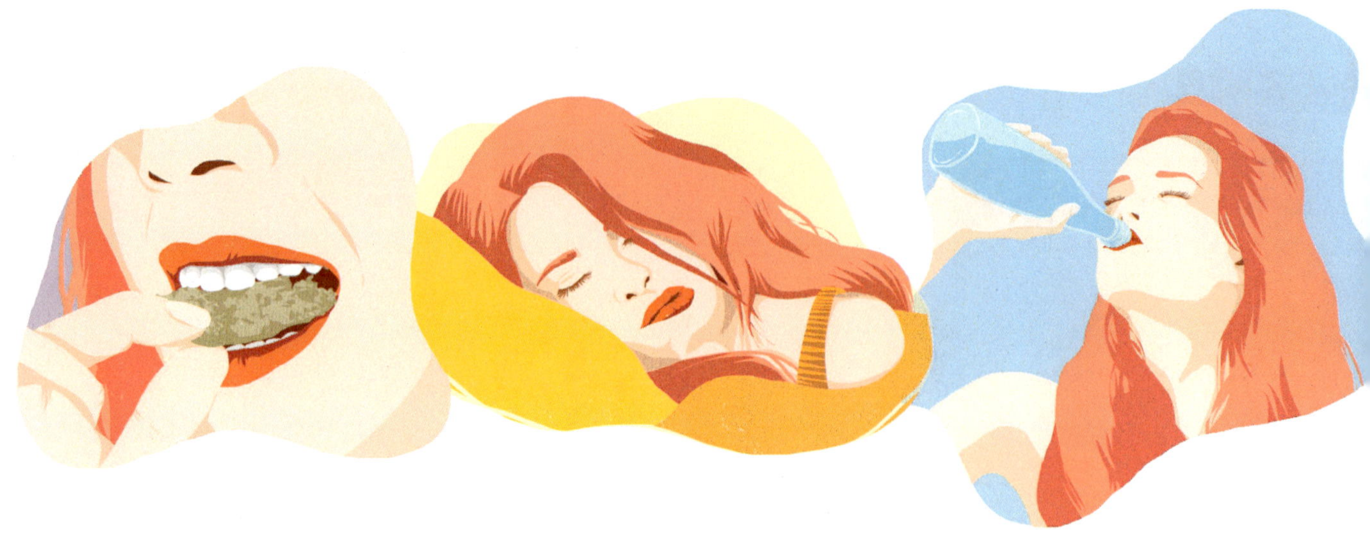

Eat well and sleep soundly

If you find yourself struggling but trapped in a circle of putting others first, consider how instigating self-care isn't just applicable in a domestic context, but is often a hallmark of great leaders. Daphna Horowitz, author, keynote speaker, and leadership coach, writes in her article, *Leaders: Put Your Own Oxygen Masks on First*: "How can you be at the top of your game if you aren't meeting your own needs first? You will only be able to provide quality guidance and support by making sure you are physically and mentally able to do so. For this, you need to be well-rested, hydrated, and ready to conquer each day with renewed energy. By refueling yourself, you're ensuring that you are giving the best version of yourself as a leader to your team."

Taking care of the basics is a theme that dominates writing on self-care and for good reason. What you eat affects your sleep, how you sleep affects your appetite, how much you drink affects both. Your body is a beautiful, complex machine whose interactive parts work both independently and in harmony with each other. Neglect one element and the rest begin to groan under the weight of bearing the load. You'll know that even one bad night's sleep can affect your decision-making process, leaving you sluggish and craving energy-laden snacks just to make it through the day.

Eat, sleep, hydrate. Three gifts you can give to yourself. Of course, you'll want to break these headings down further into subheadings. What are you eating? When? And how does your choice of food make your body feel? Choosing food that gives you sustenance and nutrition, that's the goal.

Making sleep a priority is another goal. Being deliberate about winding down for the day, creating a bedtime routine, and getting eight hours sleep, that's self-care in action. If you need any more convincing, here's Matthew Walker's stark warning on sleep deprivation from his book *Why We Sleep*: "Short sleeping increases the likelihood of your coronary arteries becoming blocked and brittle, setting you on a path toward cardiovascular disease, stroke and congestive heart failure. Fitting Charlotte Bronte's prophetic vision that a 'ruffled mind makes a restless pillow,' sleep disruption further contributes to all major psychiatric conditions, including depression, anxiety, and suicidality."

Exercise yourself . . . and your mind

Taking care of your physical needs first lights the touch paper. It leads naturally into caring for your mental and emotional needs. That time you took to go for a long walk, listen to a podcast, and be out in nature, that was taking care of your mind as well as your body. Just the act of carving out time for yourself, that's putting your oxygen mask on.

Putting aside feelings of guilt is also essential if self-care is to flourish. If going for a long run gives you back clarity of mind, helps you to fuel, hydrate, and sleep, then everyone benefits. Everyone might mean your children, your partner, your teammates, or colleagues. It might just mean your dog. But this well-rested, properly nourished version of you is nothing to feel guilty about. This version of you can give more, feel less stressed and anxious, this version of you can be the leader, parent, or partner you want to be.

Once those basics are well within your grasp, you have the power to look at what else in your life might constitute an act of self-love. How about a subscription to a movie channel, joining an online book club, or signing up to a gym class? If you know your best friend would enjoy such a gift, maybe it's time to be your own best friend. You might explore meditation, mindfulness, talk to God, write a letter, or create other daily habits that provide you with a sense of peace.

In such a time of uncertainty and fear, now is the time to take back control. Not of the world, not even of what happens today—you don't have power over any of that, but only over your own fine self. It's time to rebel against the destructive narrative of self-sacrifice. It's time to start recognizing what it is that you need to make it through this moment, with no guilt, no shame, and no limits.

RECOGNIZING YOUR EMOTIONS

When it comes to self-care, your emotional needs can be just as important as physical and mental ones. Acknowledging and accepting *all* of your emotions, even those you'd rather supress, takes effort, but being able to welcome sadness, anxiety, anger, or regret is a vital step on the path to self-love. Only when you recognize your feelings can you decide whether to change or influence them.

Next time you feel an "unwelcome" emotion, try this exercise:

Notice—simply acknowledge what you are feeling, however uncomfortable that may be, without attempting to push it away. Can you give the emotion a name? Note it here.

Accept—open your mind to the emotion and give yourself permission to feel it. Try not to judge the emotion as "good" or "bad." Simply let it be.

Examine—now start to view the emotion with curiosity. Is the emotion affecting you physically? Are your shoulders tense, or your jaw clenched? Are there different layers to what you are feeling? Jot down any thoughts.

Observe—See the emotion for what it is, a feeling that can be observed, recognized, and accepted. Can you let the emotion go?

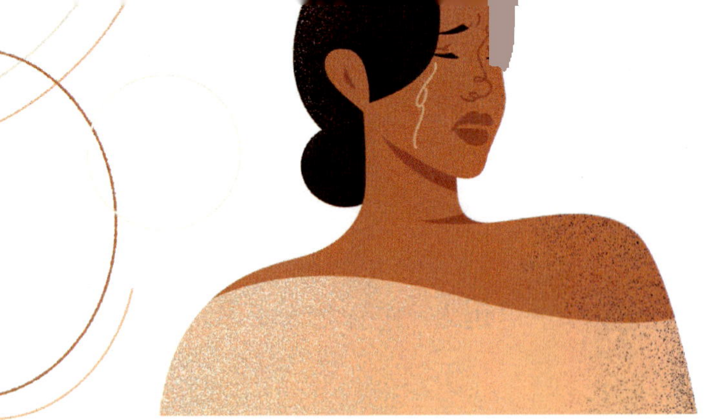
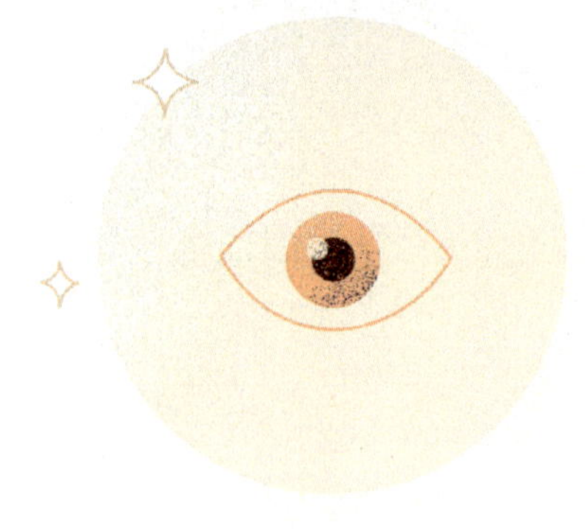

Fear of the future

Are you tired of assuming the worst is about to happen? It might be that worrying about the future is robbing you of the present

It's 7p.m. on a weekday and a loved one is late home from work. They're also not answering their phone. You immediately imagine the worst: the phone call from emergency services, a frantic trip to the hospital, rushing along the wards trying to find them, the conversation you'll have with the doctors.

Does this sound familiar? If you recognize these spiraling thoughts, you could be catastrophizing.

"Catastrophizing is an anxiety-related psychological habit or way of thinking in which the person imagines and expects the worst possible outcome of a situation, especially in the face of uncertainty," says Kimberley Wilson, a chartered psychologist and founder of Monumental Health, a clinic providing mental health care.

Catastrophizing—even the word sounds dramatic. But you don't have to be melodramatic to be a catastrophizer. Spiraling thoughts can occur in seconds and they can have a detrimental effect on psychological well-being. "At its worst, it can ramp up anxiety so much that the person can feel paralyzed and unable to function, or it may trigger a panic attack," says Kimberley.

This brings us back to that loved one who's AWOL . . . oh, and who's just strolled through the front door completely oblivious to your distress. Yes, they're late. The train was delayed for one reason or another. No, they didn't call you. Their phone had run out of power—the same reason your calls were unanswered. No emergency services, no hospital trip, no drama, but this won't prevent the same reaction the next time they or another person you care about doesn't arrive when expected.

Why do we catastrophize?

Many people who immediately hit the panic button reason that it's safeguarding, thinking it's best to prepare for the worst and be surprised when it doesn't come true. Kimberley, however, questions this. "If you habitually catastrophize, you end up living as though the worst has already happened," she cautions, "[and this] can predispose you to pessimism, cynicism, and even depression."

The tendency always to fear the worst could be rooted in a person's past. They might see it as sparing themselves from potential hurt, remembering times when they were caught offguard or frustrated by something that was unexpected, observes Kimberley. "Running through all the possible—and most terrible—scenarios in the mind can feel like an attempt to control the level of disappointment you might be exposed to."

In this instance, it's possible to take a more positive view of catastrophizing, to see it as helpful and a form of defense and protection from the worst-case scenario. Kimberley, however, points out that "in reality, all a person is doing is making themself feel bad before anything's even happened."

Is your catastrophizing out of control?

Many people experience occasions when their thoughts spiral and they imagine how difficult a task is going to be, how things will go wrong, and how they'll be left embarrassed, disappointed, or hurt. This becomes more of an obstacle when it happens frequently and starts to interfere with even the minutiae of daily life. Let's say, for example, you'd like to sit down in a café and treat yourself to a cup of coffee. It should be an effortless, enjoyable experience. But what if the very thought of buying the beverage made you think of every possible problem that might arise? Perhaps the café will be crowded and you won't be able to get a seat. What if you have to share a table with someone and you'd really rather not? What if someone nudges you and you tip your tray over? And that's to say nothing of the debate you've probably already had about the price of the coffee. How much will it cost? Is it a waste of money? Is it right to allow yourself this pleasure? As the anxiety and misplaced guilt mounts, any joy that might have been derived from the experience dissipates.

While there might be reasons behind this thought process, Kimberley feels it can be beneficial to challenge it. "To interrupt this cycle, it can be helpful first to recognize that it's not helping," she says. "It's just adding suffering to anxiety."

WAYS TO TACKLE CATASTROPHIZING

1 Look beyond the thoughts

"Try to think about the feeling that's underneath the catastrophic thoughts," says Kimberley. Are you trying to avoid experiencing certain feelings and the physical sensations they bring? Ponder what they might be. "If you can, wait them out," advises Kimberley. "Breathe slowly and they will usually pass in less than two minutes."

2 Be your best friend

Most people are their own worst critics. Sometimes it's difficult to show oneself empathy, or to think rationally. One technique of learning to talk to yourself in a logical way is to imagine you're speaking to a friend. What if they came to you with the scenario that's sparked your catastrophizing? Would you run down that road of doom with them? Or would you offer alternative routes? Try to imagine what you might say to them.

3 Write it down

Whether you keep a journal or use a notebook, when you notice your thoughts spiraling, writing it down can help. "To write about something you have to think about it," says Kimberley. "Writing is emotional processing. Writing, by hand, helps to shift a feeling into a thought, which lowers the physiological arousal, and helps to functionally reconnect the emotional centers of the brain with the rational, reasoning areas of the prefrontal cortex."

4 Accept what you cannot control

Fighting against the inevitable, something that is out of your control or you can't predict, mostly equals suffering. One approach therapists use to tackle this is called radical acceptance. It's the skill of being able to say to yourself that you cannot predict the future, and there is nothing you can do about the inevitable. Kimberley admits it takes practice, "as we all like to believe that we have more control over events [and people] than we really do," but it's an effective way of dealing with the present and future, whatever that might be.

5 Use your energy

Anxious energy can be a good thing, but try not to use it on feeling uncomfortable or overthinking. It can be employed more effectively, perhaps by going out for a walk, run, or cycle, taking up a new hobby or becoming more engaged in community projects. There are positive outlets for those pent-up thoughts and power.

6 Establish a trigger halt

The practice of mindfulness encourages the observation of thoughts without judgment and aids the return to the present moment when the mind wanders. Regular meditation practice can help you to learn how to do this. Another option is to establish a trigger to halt the spiraling process. Try saying "stop" as soon as you notice thoughts getting out of control. Whether it's out loud or in your head, it can interrupt and prevent their flow.

If you're worried about the effect your own or a loved one's tendency to catastrophize is having on your or their mental and physical well-being, it may help to see your primary care physician.

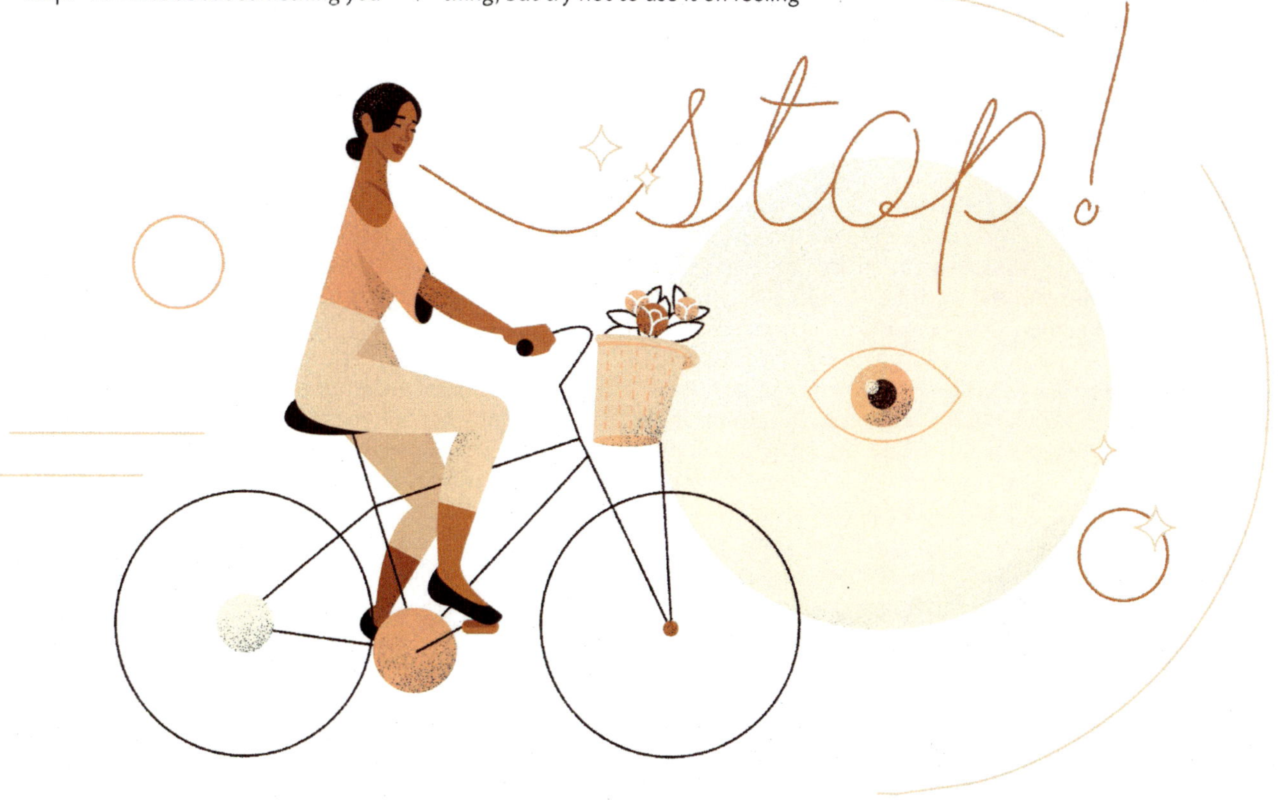

Escape into stillness

For the highly sensitive person who is fine-tuned to their environment, a regular day can quickly start to feel overwhelming. Finding stillness and tranquility requires gentle and regular self-care

Navigating life is tricky at the best of times. For those who have no choice but to feel deeply, whose minds are prone to overstimulation and who experience intense responses to people, situations, and environments, it can be even harder. The world can appear too bright, too loud, and too much to bear. One way that highly sensitive people (HSPs) can escape the noise, shake off heavy vibes, and find respite is to have access to emotional and sensory first aid. This can help to restore inner calm and instill a sense of peace.

Meaningful self-care

HSPs have no choice but to feel and experience life acutely, so using self-care tools and techniques can be helpful, but it's important to choose appropriate nurturing practices. April Snow, a holistic psychotherapist in San Francisco, believes that with the right tools and self-awareness, HSPs can thrive. In her blog at expansiveheart.com, she suggests that self-care practices need to be meaningful and centered on quiet reflection: "Quiet downtime allows our brains to process all the information we take in throughout the day and gives our nervous system time to relax. Since HSPs need their self-care to be quiet, without stimulation, it's important to think of self-care and hobbies as separate activities."

This means giving careful consideration to what constitutes quiet time and peaceful practice for the individual. This might involve more "being" than "doing" and finding gentler activities that soothe rather than stimulate. It might also mean setting boundaries with family, friends, work, or business so there's ample time to decompress from sensory overload.

Christie J. Rosen, a wellness coach, yoga instructor, and author of *Empowering the Sensitive Soul*, has always experienced life deeply, whether that's meant being sensitive to foods, fabrics, people, and smells, or highly emotionally open and aware of other people's feelings. After turning to yoga, she began to look at her health and body from a more holistic perspective. In her blog at christierosen.com, she suggests that a daily practice can help to achieve more peace and comfort in life which, in turn, makes it easier to stay grounded and centered, particularly during a challenging day.

Daily practice

"There are many practices to choose from, so the most important thing is that you find something that resonates with you and that you will commit to," says Christie. "Think of this practice as a mini-vacation. Start with 10 minutes a day and notice the shift in mind and body."

A meaningful daily self-care practice is a way of providing breathing space from an intense response to an overstimulating world. Some find it difficult to do this. They convince themselves that they don't have the time, the patience, or don't deserve the gift of self-kindness. But creating this retreat can contribute toward feeling more relaxed, peaceful, and quietly invigorated.

With a daily practice, the tools can be used to recover and sustain energy to achieve equilibrium. It can also enable HSPs to manage the frazzled times with greater ease and presence.

It's important to understand that the trait is not a personality condition or disorder. Nor is it a matter of choice. For some, it can be a burden, but there are ways it can be nurtured and managed. The idea of finding space and time for relaxation isn't to lower or remove sensitivity or sensory perception, but to provide respite from the extremes.

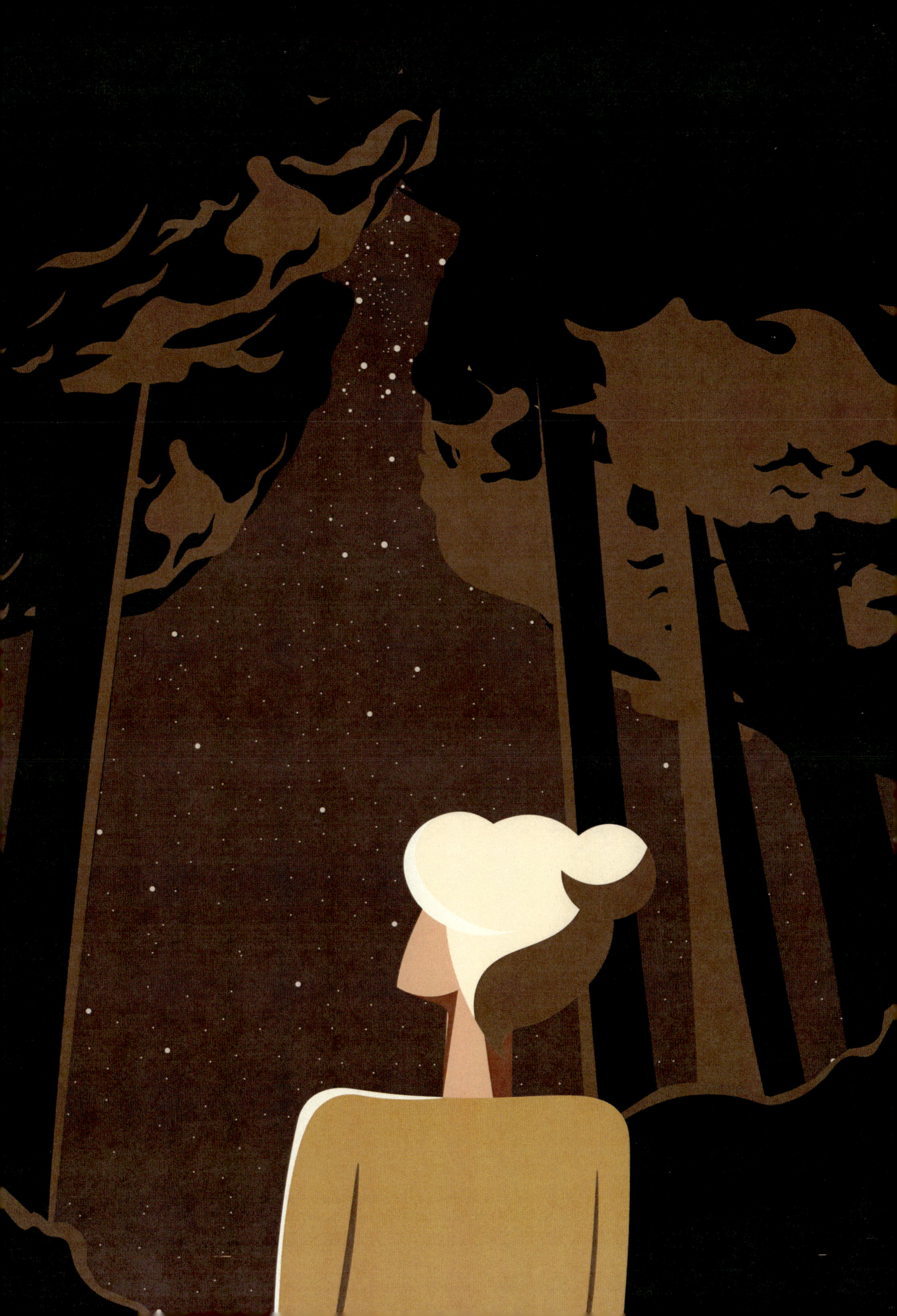

ARE YOU A HIGHLY SENSITIVE PERSON?

If you answer yes to most of these questions, it's possible that you're highly sensitive:

- ☐ Do you have a heightened reaction to or sometimes feel overwhelmed by bright lights, loud noises, powerful smells, strong tastes, coarse fabrics or textures, or electric and magnetic frequencies?
- ☐ Do you often feel the need to withdraw to somewhere quiet when life becomes hectic?
- ☐ Are you particularly emotional about people and situations?
- ☐ Do you sense, feel and take on other people's feelings, moods, and emotions?
- ☐ Do you struggle with being in a noisy, bright, or crowded place?
- ☐ Do you try to arrange your life to avoid upsetting, difficult, and overwhelming events?
- ☐ Do you have a heightened sense of the world around you?
- ☐ Are you excitable or nervous, particularly about meeting new people or embarking on fresh experiences?
- ☐ Do you seek comfort in an inner world?

Self-reflection

- What helps you become relaxed and emotionally balanced?
- Is there an activity that makes you feel lighter and more at ease? If so, what is it?
- What restful daily practice appeals to you the most?
- Where can you make time and space in your day to ease any overwhelming pressures?
- Do you need to set stricter boundaries to focus on your health and well-being?

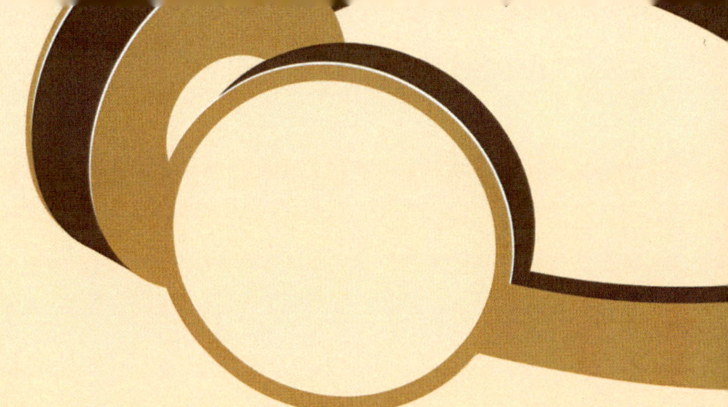

CREATE A RELAXING SELF-CARE KIT

Here are some suggestions for quiet practices that can be done every day or when others' moods or the immediate environment are taking a heavy toll. Use those that resonate with you or that you find helpful and convenient. Whether its an hour of total quiet, reading a novel while snuggled in a favorite chair, or sitting beside a babbling brook, these self-nurturing sessions can help to provide an antidote to sensory overload and stress

Calming activities

- Keep a list in your self-care kit of activities you can do to help discharge sensory overload and establish harmony. Make time for one or two of these suggestions each day.
- Create a dedicated sanctuary in your home where you can sit or lie undisturbed and slowly unwind.
- Take a solo walk in a quiet, natural place when you've completed your morning's tasks.
- Spend a few minutes alone to inhale calm and exhale tension.
- Practice tai chi, rhythmic dance, or yoga in your own comfortable space, to release pent-up energy.
- Lie or sit down in a quiet room with subdued lighting. Switch off electrical devices (you might also consider temporarily disconnecting the wifi). Meditate or use a visualization audio to let go of mind chatter.
- Listen to music that you find calming and doesn't disturb your mental stillness. It could be a gentle orchestral piece, or a recording of birdsong or waves meeting the shore.
- Stand barefoot on grass, soil, or sand to refresh and balance energy levels.
- Enjoy a hot drink. From pouring water into a mug to watching the steam rise, embrace each moment and each sip.
- Explore your thoughts and feelings in a journal. They don't have to be ordered or perfect. Use words and pictures as an outlet for reflection and expression.
- Spend time looking at photos or postcards of serene places that are meaningful to you and transport you to tranquil scenes.
- Nurture a meaningful spiritual practice.
- Sit in a chair in the garden, on a bench in a quiet park, or on a wall by the seashore. Wrap yourself in a blanket, wear clothes to match the weather, and allow the senses to settle.

Self-care kit essentials

- Notebook and pen.
- Home comforts, such as a blanket, soft pillow, or loose clothing.
- Nourishing body-care items including bubble bath, hand cream, and moisturizer. Choose unscented versions if fragrances disturb the senses.
- Earplugs and eye mask.
- Tea, or a hot drink of your choice.
- Soothing pictures, maybe landscapes or seascapes.
- Meditation and tranquil music audios.

Daily self-care benefits

- Gain space to fully relax.
- Negotiate life's ups and downs with more ease.
- Develop a deeper sense of peace.
- Have more energy for yourself and others.
- Feel calmly present and composed.
- Limit anxiety and stress.
- Be more at ease emotionally and physically.

For more information about HSPs, visit hsperson.com.

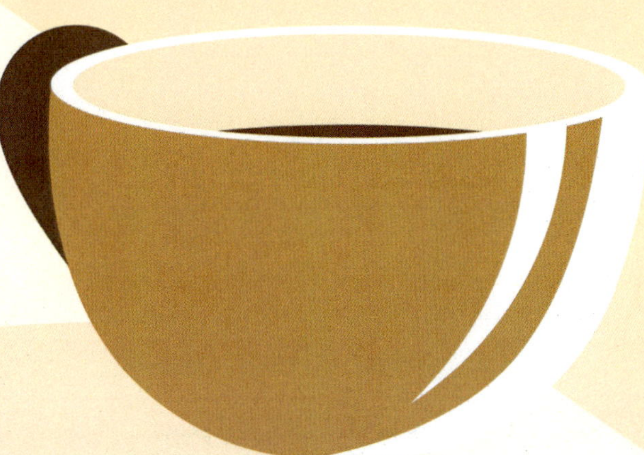

Me versus the world

It's hard when it seems that every outing, every desire, every project goes wrong and that a run of bad luck is never-ending. It can feel exhausting. But keep faith in your own ability, experience, and strength and the likelihood is that you'll see it out

Why is it that there are times when nothing seems to go right? Every decision seems to go against you, everything you do goes wrong, everything you say makes people get annoyed with you, and every idea you suggest is rebuffed. It can feel like the whole world is angrily standing around, just waiting to sabotage your every move.

Are you unlucky? Maybe. Just one of those phases? Most likely. Even though it's a phase, feeling that the world is against you can have an adverse effect on your well-being. It can make you feel lonely, anxious, and vulnerable. And it can knock your confidence as you worry about what might happen next, your decision-making, and even your character. You may ask, "Why is this happening to me?" and feel overwhelmed by the number of unfortunate events coming your way.

Your rational side knows that it's just a spell of bad luck, but when you're going through it, it can feel like a heavy burden and that time is going much slower as you wait for your fortunes to change. It might be helpful to learn that while you're going through that stage, there are strategies you can try to help bolster your mood, change your perspective, and, sometimes, gain control of the situation.

Here are a few ideas:

Be patient

You've probably heard of the phrase, "This too shall pass." As overwhelming and excruciatingly annoying as the situation is, try to remember this sentiment. The period of problems, bad luck, or issues you're facing will change. In the mind, it's easy to picture more issues arising, but if you weather the storm, the chances are that sunnier times will return. Everyone has at least one run of bad luck—sadly, it seems it's your turn now. Stay calm and be patient. Accept that this is an unpleasant time, but remind yourself that it won't last forever. You could think of it as being part of your journey and that it's happening for a reason—you just don't know what that reason is yet.

2 Believe in yourself

When you face a barrage of problems, it can knock your confidence in many ways. But you can handle any situation thrown at you, however worried you feel. Think back to when—and how—you overcame previous struggles and, more importantly, that you did overcome them. It's easy to forget when you're happy and problem-free, but draw strength from how you've coped in the past. Believe in yourself, even when you have no idea how you're going to win.

3 Assess the situation

When you're feeling more positive, you could choose to see this negative period as an opportunity for personal growth. It may sound like a cliché, but clichés are clichés for a reason. Use this time to bolster your resilience and problem-solving skills. Write down what's happened, what's going wrong, why this might be the case, how you feel about it, and how you'll try to resolve things. Exploring the situation on paper can be therapeutic and is an effective way to see situations afresh. You might work out ways to resolve any issues or even spot patterns and realize that the problems are out of your control and just a string of unlucky occurrences, or even, dare you believe it, brought on by yourself. You can take control of both how you deal with situations and how you think about them.

4 Avoid resentment

It's healthy to allow yourself to feel emotions and be upset for a while, but try not to do this for too long. You might feel resentment, that your life is unfair, but remember this is a brief period. Feeling angry with the world won't change your situation, but you can.

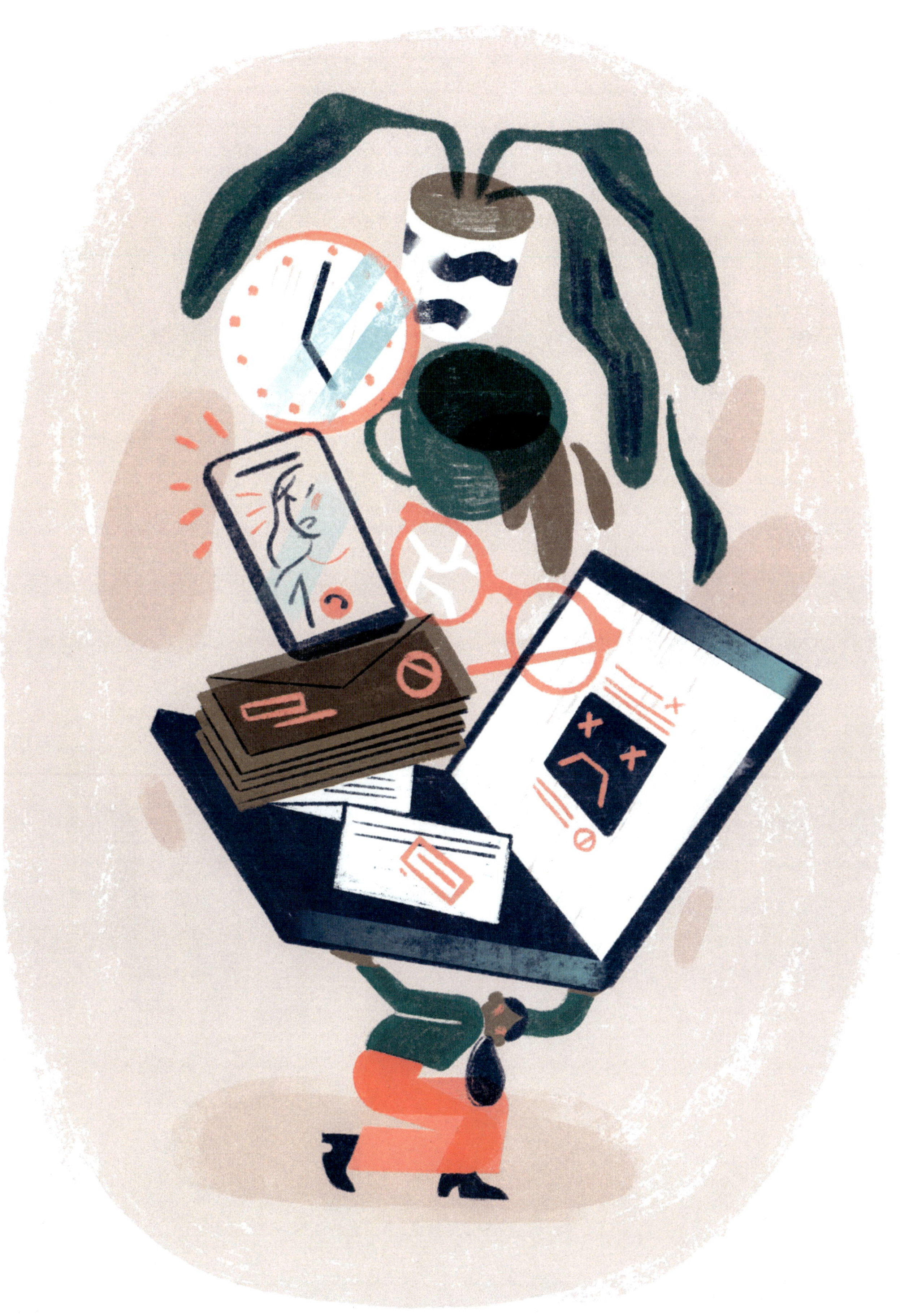

5 Seek advice

Speak to friends about what you're going through to get a different viewpoint or reassurance. They may have an insight into why things have happened or be able to suggest ways to prevent them being repeated. But what do you do when everyone is steering you away from the path you wish to take? Should you listen to them? If you truly feel you're right, you have to go with your gut. Before you do, however, speak to several people, and if those closest to you are advising you to do something different, consider why that might be the case.

6 Be wise

When things aren't going well, it can be tempting to make snap decisions that you might later regret. Think about what the happy, positive side of you would advise a friend to do in a similar situation. It's important to recognize that the feelings you have now will pass.

7 Be methodical

Try to resolve one issue at a time rather than tackling lots of difficult problems in one go. In this way, you'll be less likely to feel overwhelmed and, as things improve, more inclined to regain confidence. Visualizing future triumphs can instantly lift your mood, too, so try to hold on to the knowledge that you will soon have things to celebrate again.

8 Be creative

If you're struggling with how to resolve an issue, stop for a few hours and give your brain a break. Sometimes, solutions emerge when you're being creative. With the issues in your mind, write a poem or story and see what ideas are raised from your subconscious. Try listening to music, reading, gardening, painting, drawing, or meditating and see what ideas emerge. These exercises can also help with anxiety about the spell of bad luck.

9 Accept that life is unpredictable

Alongside all the happiness and positive experiences in life, the world will always throw unexpected and unpredictable challenges in your way. They aren't always bad. And there may even come a time when you look back and can draw strength from what happened.

10 Positive outlook

Choose positive, optimistic but honest people to spend time with. You might not want to talk about your problems, but just need a break from thinking about them, and this can be hugely beneficial. See your loved ones, spend time with people of all ages and do things that give your mind a break, whether that's watching a movie, exercising, reading, or doing a crossword. Looking at the positives in life can give things a broader perspective. This isn't always easy when everything seems to be going wrong—and it doesn't negate or undermine your current anxiety or hurt—but it might help you to cope with the inclement weather. And remember that after the storm comes the rainbow.

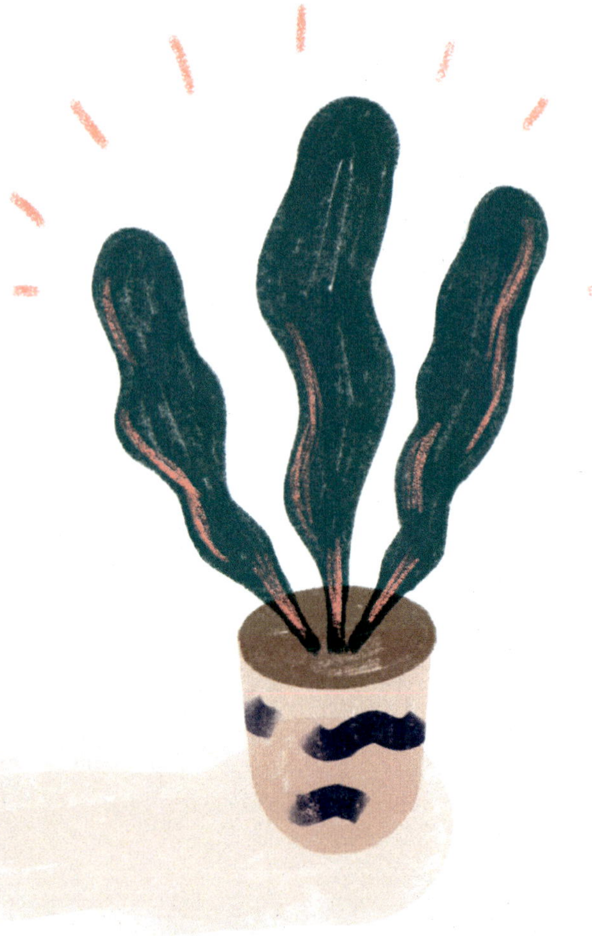

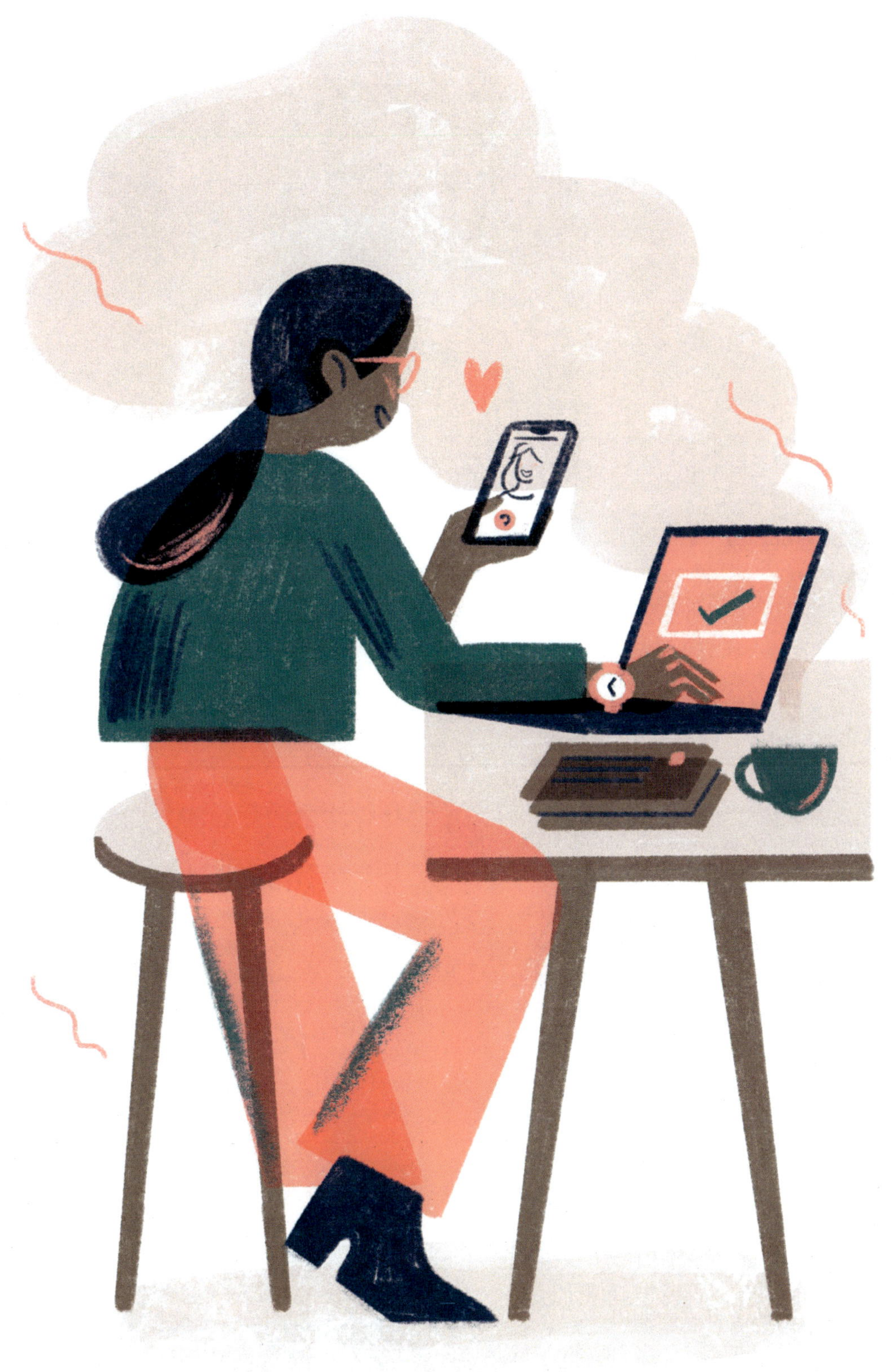

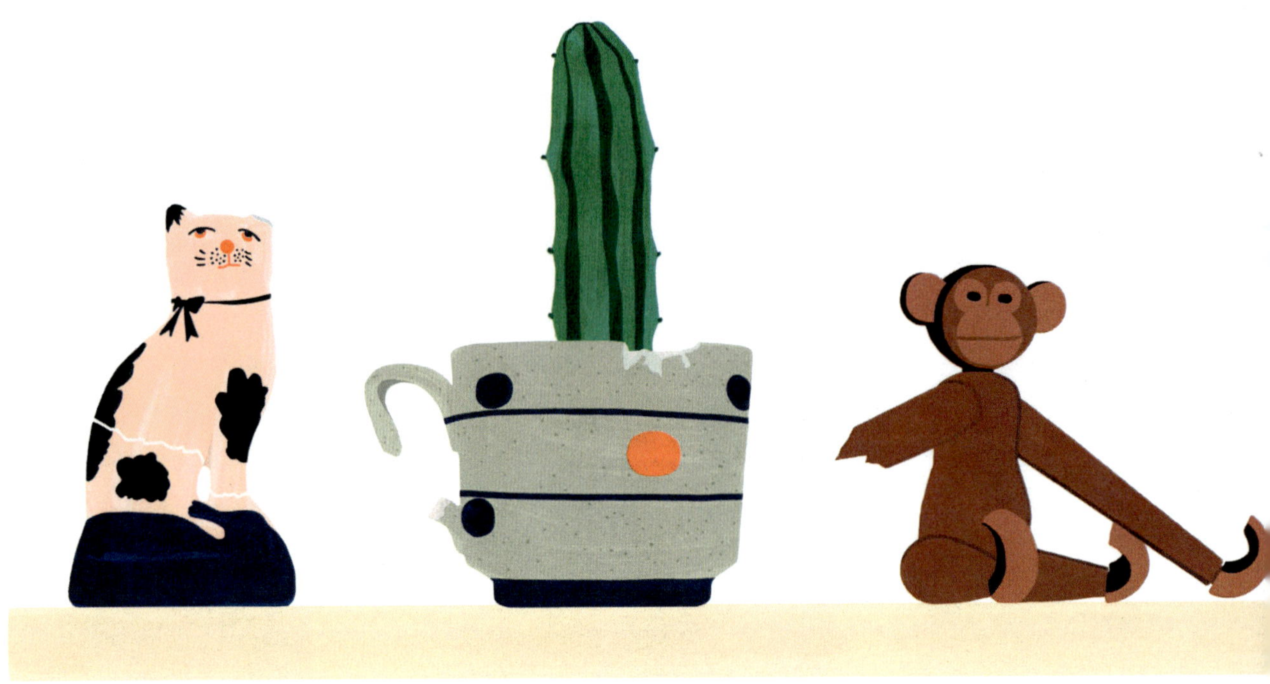

Fresh perspective

Many strive to hide or remove character traits deemed less than perfect, but is there another way to look at them—one that embraces and celebrates humanity in all its guises?

From lifestyle coaches to online therapy, these days there are increasingly more ways to help you to help yourself, to fix those parts of your character that are deemed "less than perfect." Advice is just a click away, and it seems there's no excuse for quirks of personality to remain unchecked. Coping with life or getting support to deal with past hurts is no longer enough. Now, turning to therapists for self-improvement, to become a better version of yourself, is the choice of today's self-aware citizen.

Desire for change

Rebecca Lockwood, a neurolinguistic programming (NLP) coach and author, knows this all too well. Over the past few years, she's noticed that her clients' reasons for seeking help have shifted, particularly when it comes to changing themselves, in the desire for greater business success.

"People used to want to feel more confident, so they could do public speaking, for example," says Rebecca. "Now, it's more often the case that people are wanting to gain more confidence to become more visible, which to them means in their personal brand, in their business. They want to do more video and put themselves out there on social media, without worrying about what other people think of them."

This move away from objective goal to personal goal marks a shift in people's desire for better personal branding, in both their professional and personal lives, particularly when played out through the lens of social media. Setting up that carefully lit vacation photo, the happy family unit, or the most exquisite looking meal can also be seen as examples of personal branding.

While life through this lens often does look perfect, what is it that drives you to deny the imperfections that make you unique? Not the bad habits, the chronic lateness, or talking over people to get your voice heard loudest, but the real, human elements of what makes you, you.

Take Sam, for example, a 38-year-old father of two. Throughout his life, Sam has struggled with traits of obsessive-compulsive disorder. When he was younger they worried him, and even when he married he kept them from his wife for as long as he could. They weren't extreme, but they were ritualized—a certain order that had to be kept. During moments of stress, these traits would be particularly compelling. Not a fan of enclosed spaces, Sam would run through his own checklist in his head before stepping inside an elevator. Once inside and heading up or down, he would go back through that checklist, reciting it silently, right up until the elevator doors slid back open, to his great relief.

Focus on the positive

For many, having these same traits wouldn't be something to talk about, and certainly not something to be celebrated. Some would perhaps seek treatment for them. But for Sam, denying this so-called flaw in his character would be to deny a major part of himself. His attitude to this element

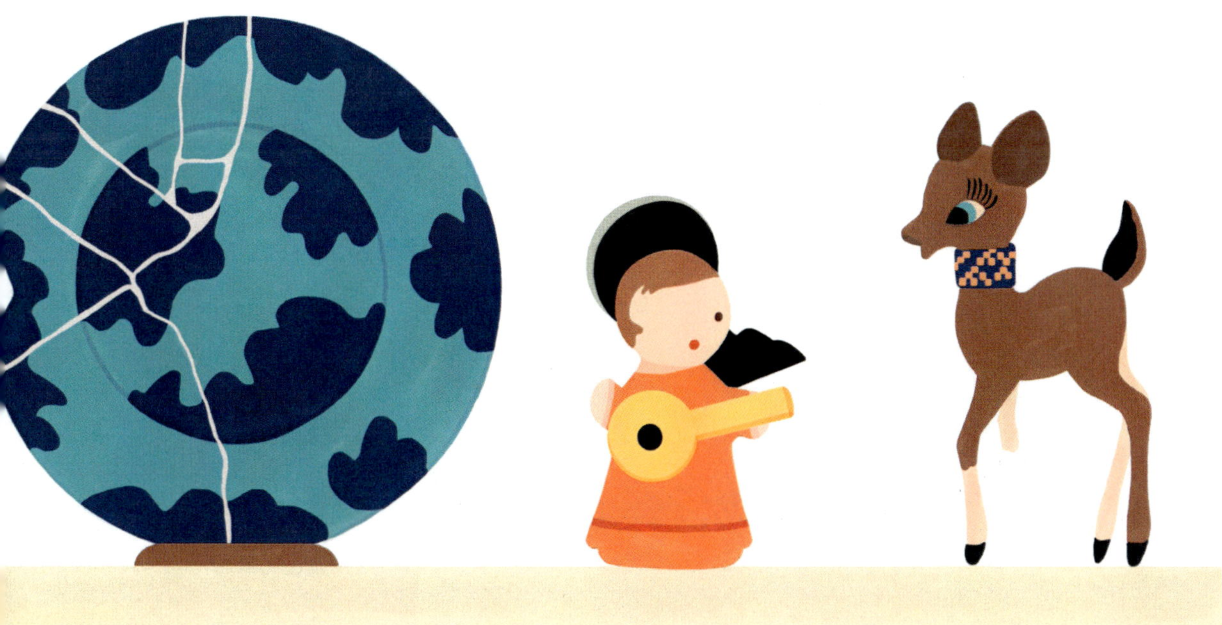

of his personality has undergone significant changes over the years: "When I was really young, I felt like I had a superpower," he says. "I could make things happen by thinking about them hard enough or following a sequence in my thoughts. When I got a bit older and learned more about OCD, I became ashamed and worried about what people would think of me.

"I think now that I'm more experienced and more secure in myself, this element of my personality is, again, more like a superpower. It helps me. It gives me order and it helps me to focus. For example, in the morning I get ready for work in a very specific order and at the same time every day. If I didn't do it that way, I'd forget something, especially in the hustle and bustle of my house in the morning. I embrace my OCD traits and I let them work for me, not against me."

Another point of view

Other so-called imperfections can be viewed though a fresh pair of eyes. Even therapists sometimes need to learn this lesson about themselves. Rebecca remembers the moment that she realized her imperfections were not necessarily a "bad" thing, and could be a force for good in her professional life.

"I do so much work on myself, to not judge myself or my imperfections," she says. "My book, *Step into your Personal Potential*, is all about checking in with yourself and loving yourself whole. One of the things that I used to believe was an imperfection of mine is that I love to do a lot of things—I am very creative and I quickly do projects and then move on.

"It was when I released this particular book that I realized how much of an asset it is. When I had the idea, I was eating dinner at my kitchen table with my mom and two children. As soon as I'd eaten, I ran upstairs and started working. I worked solidly on the book for two weeks, released it within a month and became a bestselling author for the second time."

It's worth looking at where notions of imperfection come from and how differences in personality can end up carrying such negative values. Perhaps, for some people, the idea that there are undesirable aspects of their personality is a concept that's been driven home since childhood, or it might stem from a non-supportive romantic partner or, like Sam, from having a brain that works differently from what's considered normal.

Find self-acceptance

Rebecca believes that, for many people, it comes from a lack of self-acceptance and an inability to fully appreciate yourself for who you are, warts and all. Learning to do this and embracing your imperfections marks the beginning of being able to move forward with your life.

"We can get so caught up in wanting to be a certain way and have certain things," she says. "It's more important to love yourself fully, as you are. The aim isn't to change you—it's to not care about the imperfections in the first place, not give them a negative meaning or attach judgment toward yourself for feeling as though there's imperfection there."

If it's possible to find a sense of neutrality toward your imperfections then that's surely a starting point toward a fuller acceptance of who you are. While others may press you to change or, worse, attempt to reduce you, the pressure to do away with those allegedly less-than-perfect features often comes directly from within—from you.

In a world where the presentation and idea of perfect often comes at the expense of reality, maybe it's time to embrace the messiness, the fun, and, yes, the frustrations that come from being a whole person. A person with talents, desires, and ambitions, and with imperfections that are complicated, brilliant, and uniquely you.

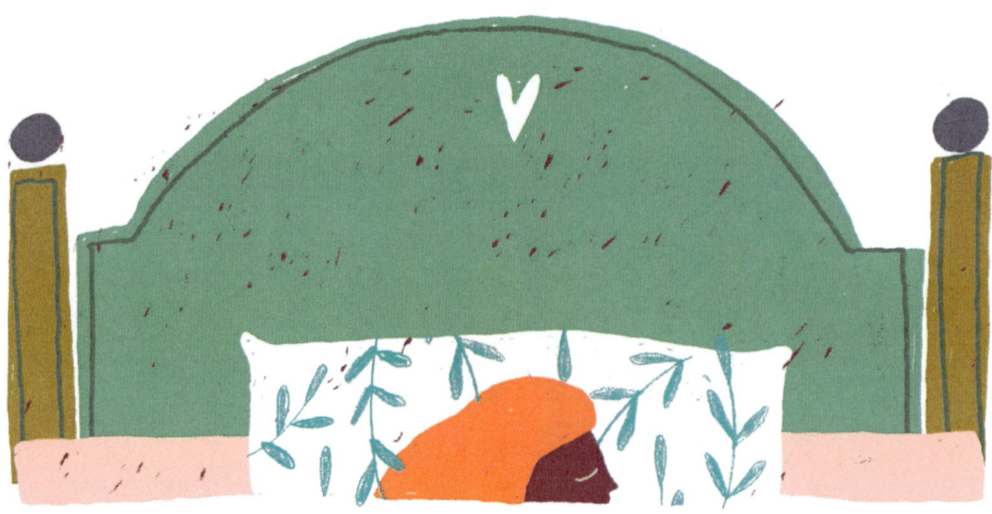

Forever strong?

When you're the person everyone always turns to for advice and emotional support it can be hard to admit if you're feeling overwhelmed, low, or worried. Yet being open and honest at these moments could be beneficial all round

It can feel rewarding to be approached for advice. When someone values your time, your listening ear, and your take on things, when they trust you enough to share their thoughts or concerns with you—well, who wouldn't feel validated by that? As troubling as the other person's issues might be, it's not unusual to feel good about being the person they turn to.

And rightly so because being trusted by others speaks volumes about a person. It demonstrates magnetism and sagaciousness, an aura of calm, strength, and good sense. People who combine these qualities are often natural leaders. Even if they're not sparkling with obvious charisma, their empathetic nature gives them a different kind of attractiveness.

Role reversals

Do you know someone like this—or are you perhaps that person? And what happens when someone who's always there for everyone else needs someone to be there for them? One might suppose that everyone who's previously benefitted from the strong person's support might rally around to return the favor, but although this is sometimes the case, there's often a flip side to being the strong one. It can be isolating. Hang on—how can this be when the person to whom everyone turns in a crisis is magnetic, a natural leader?

A downside to being someone to whom people look up is that signs of fallibility can shake the status quo. Individuals who are accustomed to having a particular colleague, friend, or family member to lean on may feel awkward and unsure when that person expresses need or demonstrates vulnerability. When roles are reversed, it can create feelings of deep discomfort. This also applies to people who usually appear to have it all together—when someone always plays a strong role, it can feel hard to admit that something's on their mind. Because so much of how people perceive themselves is bound up with how others see them, expressing emotions or acting out of character may shake their own sense of identity, as well as sparking worry about how they'll be viewed externally. Once they step out of character, will they ever be able to assume that role again? And if not, who will they be then?

Hero to zero

A high school principal, for example, is generally seen as a figure of authority by their students. They're perceived as rule-abiding and in control. Imagine, then, if this same principal were to front an assembly in pajamas, saying their anxiety was so overwhelming that morning that they could barely face getting out of bed?

It's an extreme example, and obviously one that relates to a professional, rather than personal, relationship, but it illustrates the point: Once the cape of authority has been cast off, how easy is it to assume it again? How would the students feel and react? Would they rush forward with offers of help? Would they applaud their principal's honesty? Would they stifle mocking laughter? Or would they sit in disbelieving silence?

Chances are it would be one of the last two responses. It's difficult—for both parties—when someone who's always

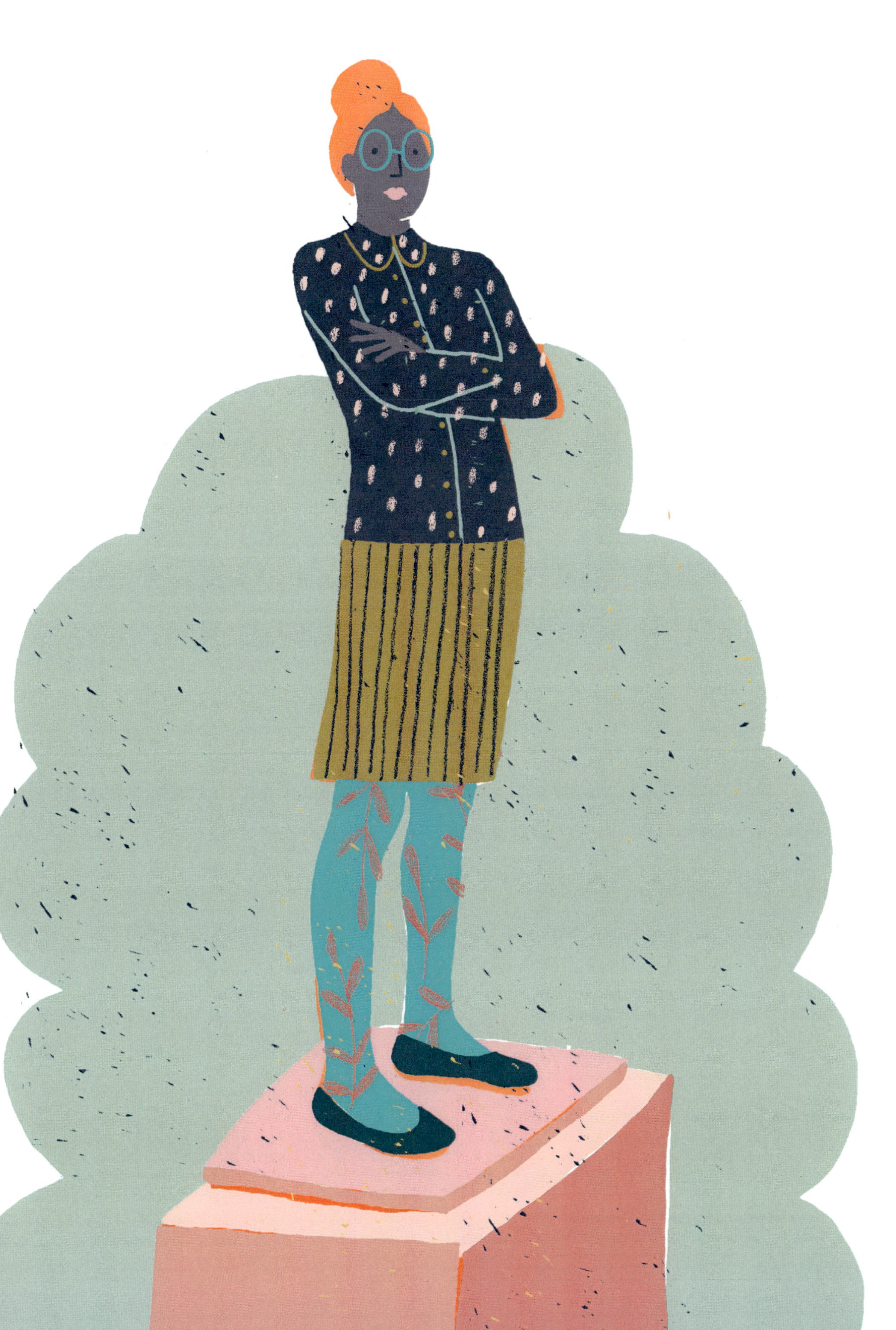

"The world breaks everyone, and afterward, some are strong at the broken places"

ERNEST HEMINGWAY, A FAREWELL TO ARMS

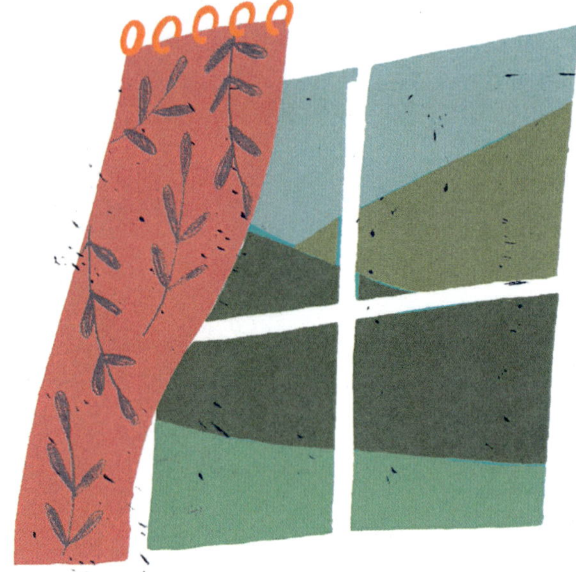

"the strong one" needs help. In families, these shifts occur naturally in parent/child relationships. As the years go by, the parent ceases to be all-powerful and children often take on helping and caring roles, which can be challenging for both sides.

Great expectations

It's something of a double-edged sword when people have high hopes of others. On the one hand, it's lovely to be thought well of—who wouldn't prefer to hear "I know you'll knock them dead at that job interview," rather than "Hmmm, I really can't see you getting that role"? On the other hand, appreciation and encouragement often come with pressure and nerves: "Oh no! What if I don't get the job? What will everyone think?"

When people don't manage to live up to a certain expectation, comments such as "I can't believe it. I really thought you had that one in the bag" can feel more like disapproval, or a rebuke, than a supportive statement of allegiance. If you take this example and apply it to always seeming in control it's possible to see how the expectation of strength may actually add to a sense of crisis, causing the strong one to internalize their feelings of fear or anxiety in case sharing them elicited responses such as "I'm so surprised. I always thought you were so strong."

Spread the load

It's helpful to foster a range of relationships in which each individual has the space to assume different mantles. Even the most successful high school principal has to defer to some form of governing body—and, with any luck, has people in their personal life with whom they can relax and, yes, even wear pajamas.

It may be that a strong-one role exists within the family. Perhaps years of mediating between parents and siblings has made it difficult to be anything but the person everyone turns to in a crisis. It may feel there's no space to admit to one's own feelings of upset or worry, that all available airtime is taken up by everyone else.

When family ties are oriented along these lines, it's important that more equal relationships exist outside of the family. If close friends seem constantly to be taking far more than they're giving, then it might be helpful to seek out people with whom more equally weighted relationships can be built and nurtured.

Redrawing the lines

That's not to say that the status quo must be accepted when it comes to relationships and the give and take of emotional support within them. As uncomfortable as it may feel to admit fragility, it's important for personal health, as well as the health of the relationship.

Begin, perhaps, by occasionally saying "no" when someone starts to unload. It may feel uncomfortable, but you could respond by saying: "I'm really sorry, but I have a lot going on at the moment and I'd hate not to give you the support you need. I hope you'll be okay—perhaps there's someone else you can talk to?"

Being accustomed to being there for everyone else can make saying "no" feel awkward, but it's critical everyone takes some responsibility for where they are in their relationships. The habit of saying or implying "yes" to requests for help and support needs to be nipped in the bud for equilibrium to be created and restored.

Alternatively, try referring to personal problems without delving into the details. For instance: "I'm sorry, I can't be there for you right now, but my father has been sick and I'm worried about him," or "I'm up against a huge deadline at work and it's taking up all of my time and energy." A non-elaborate statement might help to stop in their tracks someone who was about to offload their woes. It could also prompt a response of help, with the person asking if there's anything they can do.

Such admissions are signs of being human. One aspect of always being the strong one is that it's easy to start believing in one's own superpowers, but small acknowledgments that everyone has tricky times can assist people on both sides of the equation.

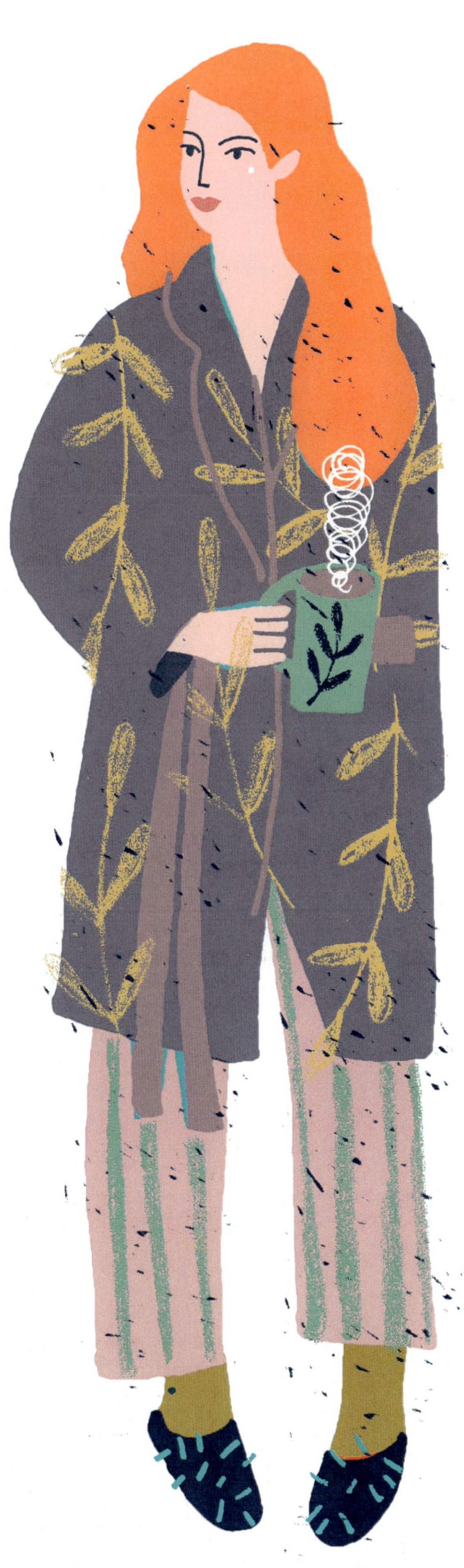

PEDESTAL OR STATUE?

Some people fall more naturally into the role of supporter, and some into the role of supported, but that's not to say that's the only thing they're capable of being

Always the pedestal?

If being the sounding board for everyone else's problems is adding to feelings of being overwhelmed, or contributing to a sense that being the ears means never being permitted to be the mouth, then there's a danger of becoming drained and depleted, unable to care for oneself, let alone anyone else.

- Take a break from attending occasions that give rise to moth-to-flame scenarios (with you being the latter).
- Be honest in low-key, comfortable ways. You don't need to say: "I'm having a nightmare time." You could reply: "I know, right? Things can get tricky—for me too, right now. I hope we can both get things straightened out."
- Remember that people who can't be there for you when you have a hard time aren't unworthy of your love. It's more that they need to be balanced out with other people and relationships.

Always the statue?

- Take a hard, honest look at your pedestal. Might there be cracks, however imperceptible, in it? No pedestal can support multiple statues.
- Try not to be self-absorbed. Whatever the outward appearance of the statue—check in with them.
- Be sure not to make one person the ears for every problem. Needing to offload is fine, but talking to different people about relationships, work, or personal worries may ensure adequate support without anyone having to feel overwhelmed.

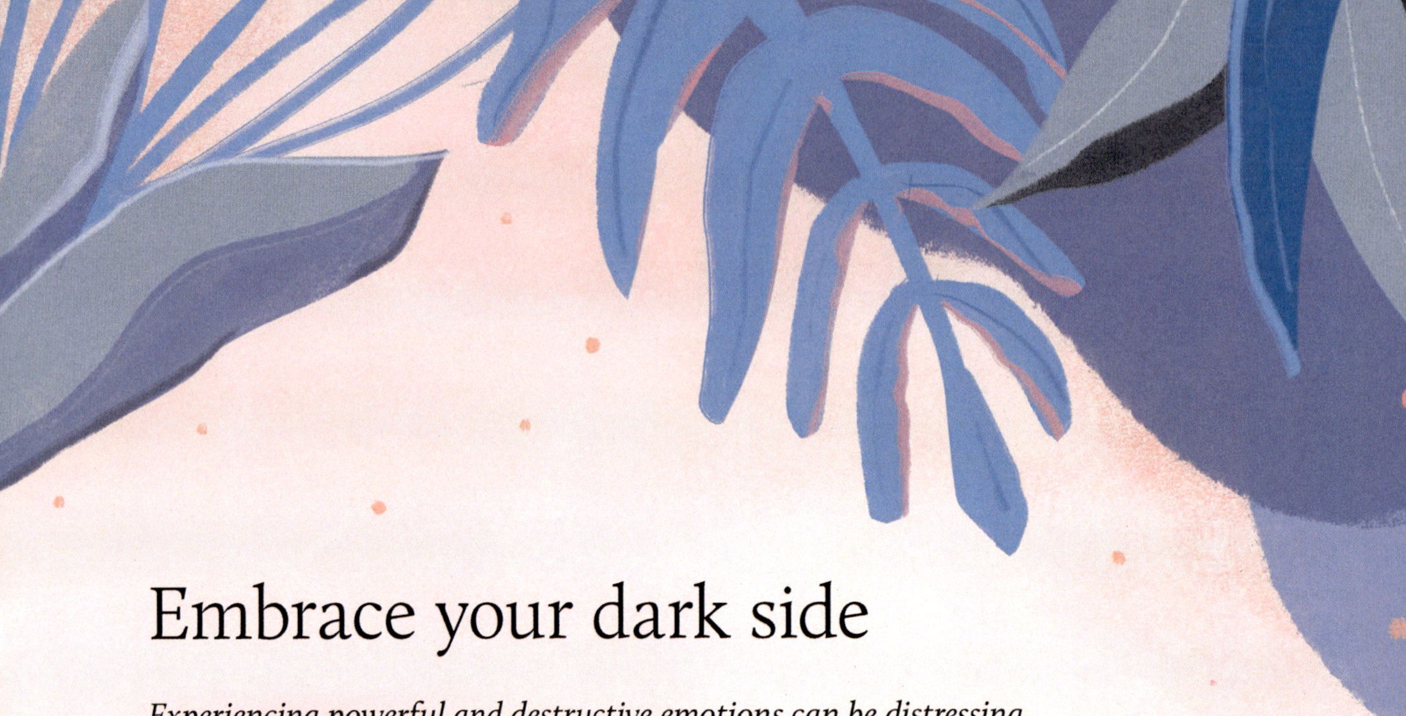

Embrace your dark side

Experiencing powerful and destructive emotions can be distressing. Here's how to begin to live alongside them

Most people have been derailed by their emotions at some point. Perhaps it was seeing a partner talking to their ex, hearing that a friend had been promoted, or being on the receiving end of a rude sales assistant. Before you know it a torrent of emotional force has been unleashed and you find yourself sat there in the aftermath wondering what happened.

Getting pushed around by strong emotions isn't unusual. Fear, jealousy, greed, or rage are some of the big ones that burst through the floodgates and leave a trail of destruction. While it can seem counterintuitive to do anything but try to eradicate them from your life (or else put them in a corner of your mind and bolt the door), this can be more detrimental. When you get to know and even take care of destructive emotions, your relationship with them can begin to transform.

What does a destructive emotion look like?

For some, these emotions might be externally focused, blaming the world and those around them for injustices or things that have gone wrong. For others, they are targeted internally, for example, berating yourself over a failure, or for your appearance. They can lead people to isolate themselves, use substances to cope, or else use loved ones as metaphorical punchbags. The telltale signs can be the strength of the emotion; denial of its existence; not taking responsibility for the situation; feeling afraid or ashamed of having the emotion; and seeing disruption at home, work, and with friends and family as a result.

For Jane Kirby, a former PR director, anxiety caused destruction in her life. She says: "I started to lose interest in my work. I felt distant from my colleagues and eventually I walked away from my business as I couldn't see a way forward. I couldn't function and it had a massive impact on my husband, even though he was there for me."

Powerful, destructive emotions can arise with such force that it can feel like they blazed in from out of the blue with zero notice. Claire*, a marketing manager, says: "My anger can feel like it comes on so suddenly and ends up in an outburst. There's just so much inside that feels like it needs to come out." The triggers for such emotions are often small, but they may have been slowly building over time. Is it speaking with a particular person that evokes the feeling? Being in a certain setting? Or every time the topic turns to why you haven't found a partner, settled down, had a family, or got a "real" job? Uncovering your own triggers can help you to understand the emotion and even preempt outbursts. Look out for early physical warning signs that your mood is changing (think tightened muscles and jaw, changes in your breathing, shoulders starting to tense, becoming hotter). The body often shows the first subtle signs of changing emotions, so becoming more attuned with physical responses is important.

It's understandable to say that you don't want to feel hatred, jealousy, or anxiety. Wouldn't life be easier without them? The truth, however, is that they're hardwired into the brain at a core, visceral level to aid survival. To eradicate them is both impossible and unwise. What you can learn to do is respond to them in a different way so that you see them for what they are and find healthy ways to release them. It is in fact the pushing away, the denial, and the subsequent shame and guilt that can keep destructive emotions in play. Having an unpleasant or challenging

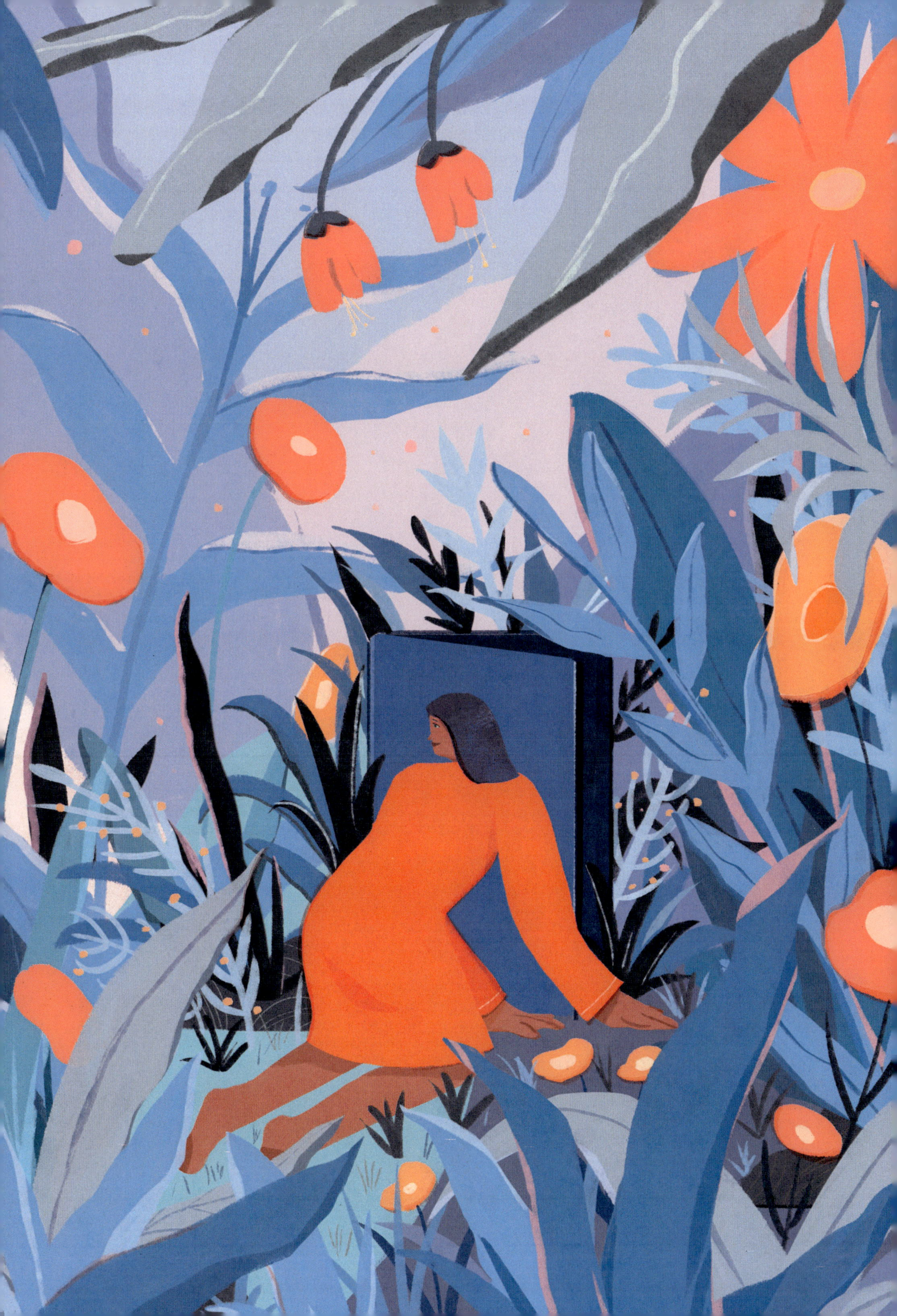

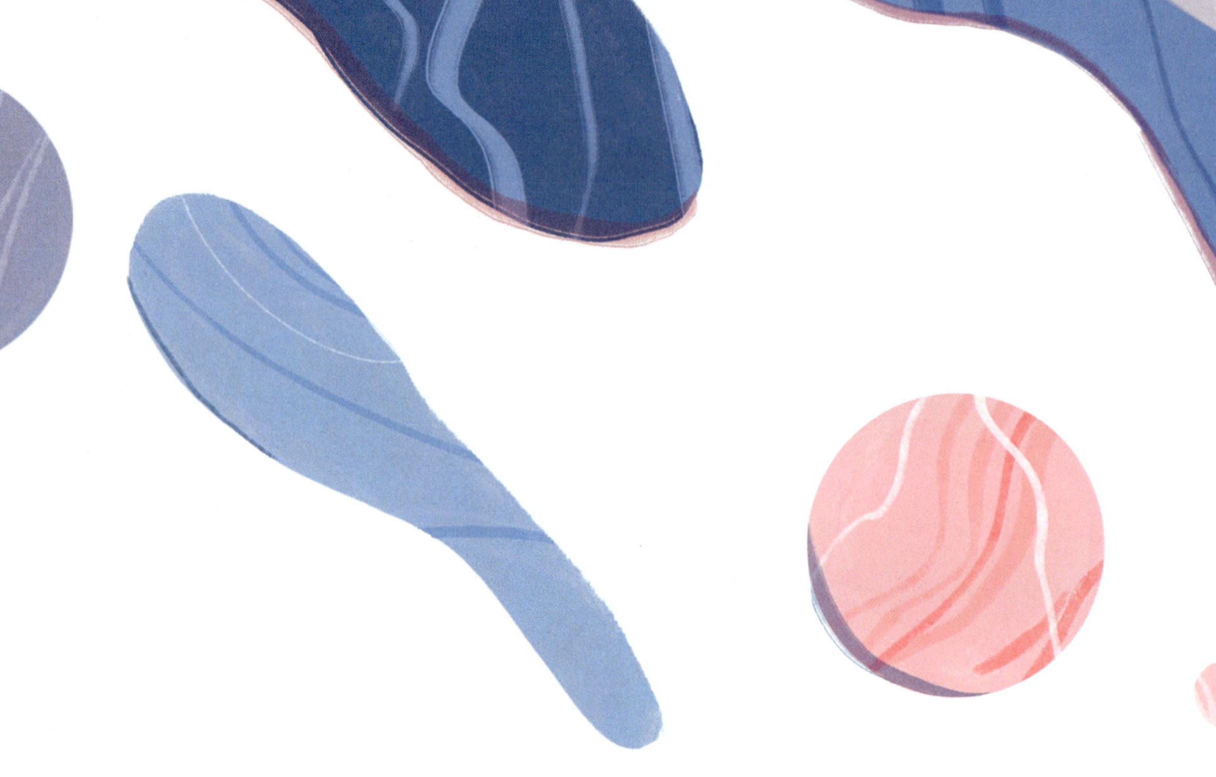

emotion is not in itself necessarily the issue, it is when you cannot bring any level of acceptance to what you are experiencing, as well as the resulting behavior that follows the emotion. Claire says: "I used to avoid dealing with stress and anger and go out drinking and partying as a quick fix, but it wasn't sustainable. Trying to cope like this ended up causing more problems, like not having any energy at work and getting into the wrong relationships."

Without pushing away your most challenging emotions you can gently start getting to know them. How strong is it (rating from zero to 100 percent)? Where does it show up in your body? What does it make you want to do? It can even be helpful to try to draw or write about a difficult or destructive emotion, perhaps seeing what it might look like as a person or animal, even what color it might be. Once you have registered its presence, you can try receiving the message with gratitude (thank you brain for letting me know I feel jealous around my partner, I know I need to strengthen our relationship to feel more secure). You can then direct your attention to a healthy, absorbing task such as tackling the problem itself, calling a friend, or going for a walk. Claire found exercise helpful: "Running has been the only thing that has really cut through the stress. It's easy not to bother but I feel empowered afterward and I'm generally a nicer person to be around."

Activities that engage the senses are useful, perhaps using essential oils to massage your hands, running a warm bath, sipping a warm drink, doing some gentle yoga or breathing exercises. This time spent tending to your own needs helps engage the parasympathetic system meaning you feel more relaxed and are no longer functioning in fight-or-flight mode.

While it's possible to understand how negative emotions can lead to destruction, what about those traditionally viewed as pleasant or positive? It's not unusual for those who have had difficult experiences in relationships to act out when closeness and affection is encountered, often with an underlying fear of being abandoned or losing themselves. Being kind to yourself can also feel dangerous and unfamiliar, particularly as in Western society this can feel indulgent and self-important.

There will be times where you lose control of your emotions as well as days when the distress is so great that to start to face them on your own may be overwhelming. The first incidence requires letting go of self-criticism and accepting that you are a human being who doesn't always get things right. The latter might require a discussion with your family doctor or another supportive professional who can work with you to look at managing destructive emotions and behaviors. Jane found that there was a way back to her old self from anxiety and says: "I began to realize that there was a key that would unlock the door to my suffering and bring healing. For me it was the support of friends and family, medication, a brilliant doctor, counseling, and prayer."

It can be helpful to think about life like a jigsaw puzzle with various shades of dark and light pieces, all essential in making up the whole picture. If you throw away the dark pieces the picture no longer makes sense, and this is the same in your life. It's only when you learn how to live with, and look after, the more challenging and destructive parts of yourself can you hope to stumble upon your true greatness. As poet and scholar Rumi said: "The wound is the place where the light enters you." This can be a powerful reminder not to shy away from difficult emotions, but to turn toward them to move forward with life.

*If you need further support, please see your primary care physician. *Name changed.*

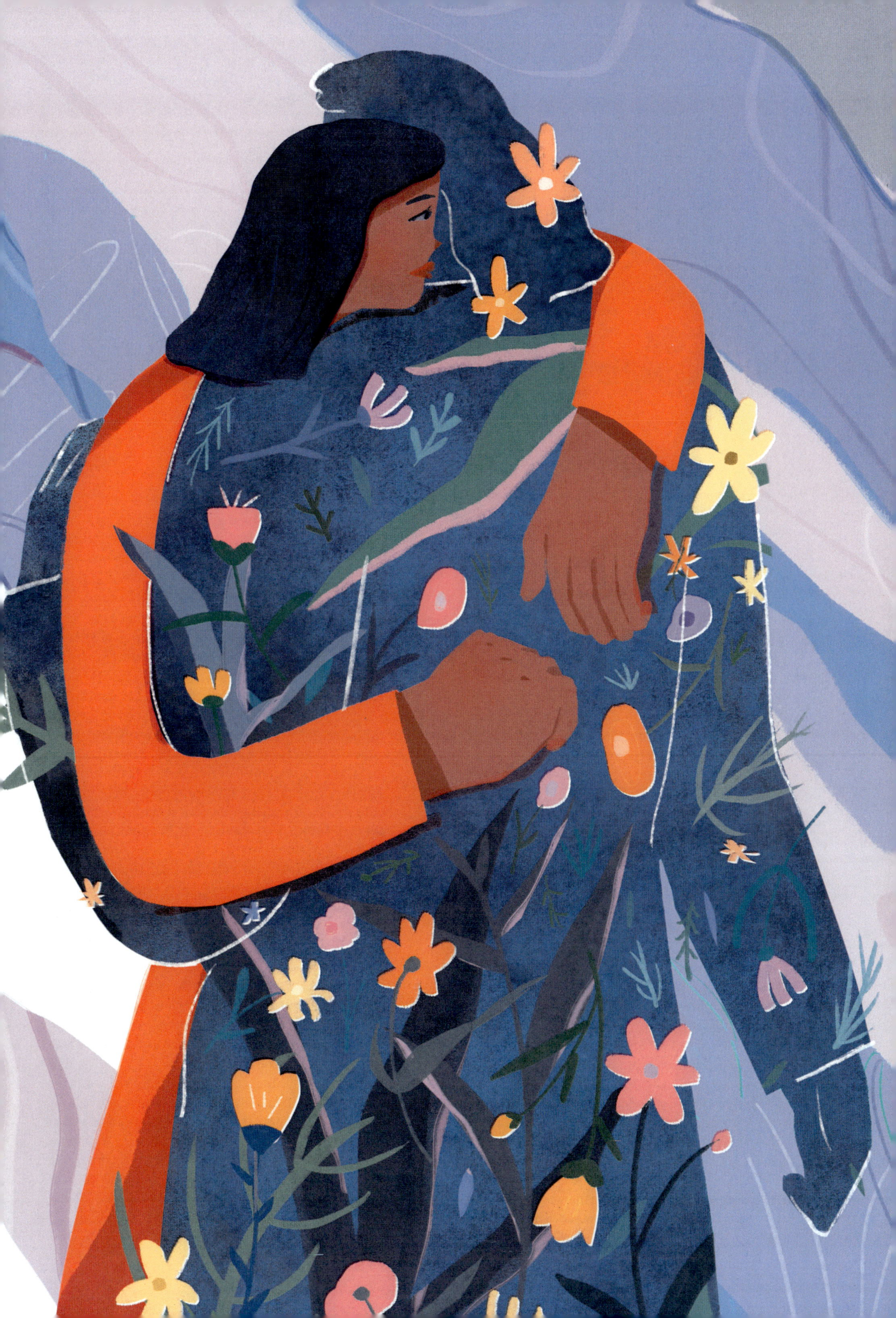

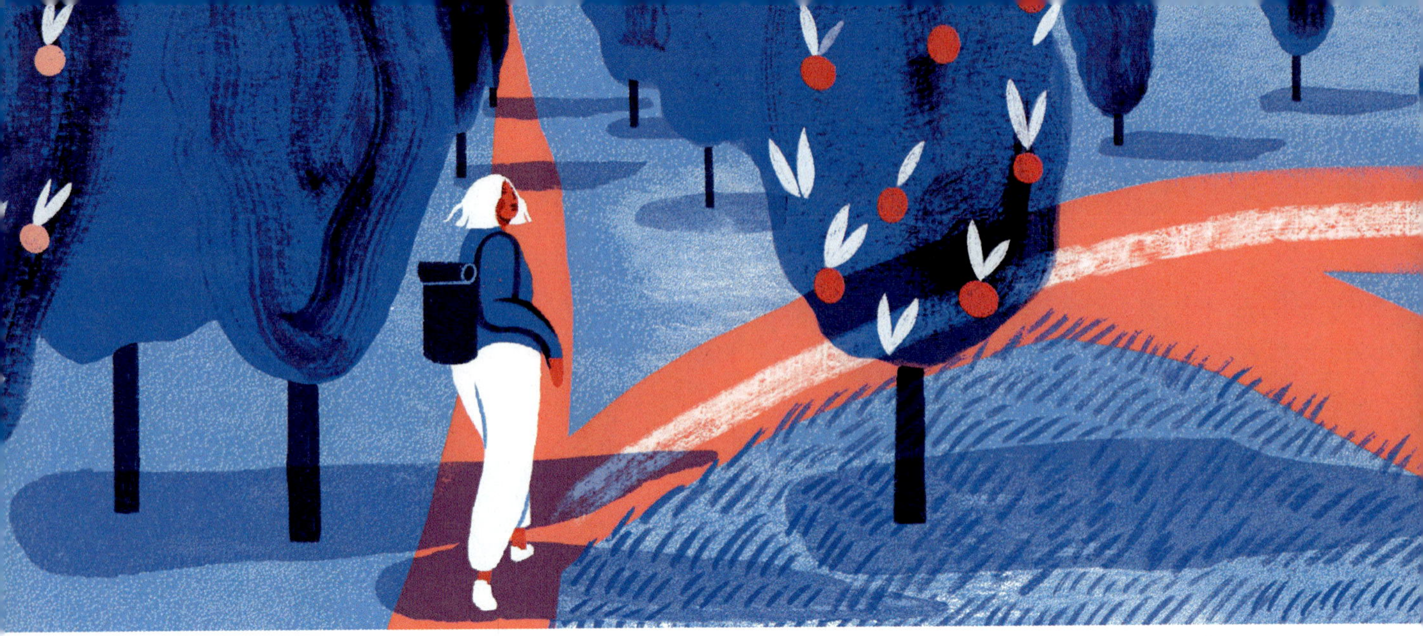

No limits

Feel stuck in a groove you don't like? It might be you need to explore what's keeping you there in order to make the changes that will lead you toward the life you really want

If you're waking up each day feeling discontented with life—be it because you're working in a job you don't like, you've settled in a place that feels soul-destroying, or you're existing (perhaps even comfortably), while sensing you're not where you want to be—it can seem near impossible to believe and trust that anything will change. In your mind, the situation might feel static, your options restricted, your path to fulfillment blocked. But these are limiting thoughts that can stop you from seeing that change is possible. One way to alter this perception is to realize there are choices. And the first one could be to cast off the thoughts, feelings, and habits that are blocking your route to personal happiness and contentment.

Let go of your fears

This doesn't mean it's easy, however. Changing your outlook and overriding deeply rooted thoughts and beliefs can be a struggle. Puja K. McClymont is a neuro-linguistic programming mindset, life, and business coach, who helps people find confidence and gain more control of their lives. "Nearly anything to do with change is connected with fear and the actual fear of making changes," she says. "We are creatures of habit, yet we tend to want so much more from our lives without making the changes necessary to achieve them."

These negative, fear-fueled beliefs tend to run over and over in a loop and can keep people where they are, hostages to their own limiting thoughts and ideas. This can deter them from trying fresh avenues, following their intuition, and exploring options that might be more fulfilling. A person's mindset can easily be influenced by environment, circumstances, experiences, and other people's beliefs. That person then creates a story for themselves that is based upon these influences. If the mindset is fueled by an undercurrent of fear, this is likely to keep a person stuck but safe, constrained but comfortable, and they can end up existing rather than living. Holding on to this mindset fortifies the life you don't want, and it can become weighed down by heavy layers of restrictions, sadness, and regret. Given permission, self-limiting thoughts can create a jail and keep you in there for life.

Kitty Waters, a transformational teacher, host of a podcast called Kitty Talks and cocreator of The Network for Transformational Leaders, is on a mission to help people improve their lives. Her Do Your Dharma course helps people to find their true calling, which involves letting go of feeling stuck and creating a positive mindset that's in alignment with the life they want.

Kitty says: "Awareness is the first step to change. Everything is energy. What you focus on expands, and where energy goes, focus flows. You shape your life experience through your beliefs, and your thoughts and words create your reality. When you're aware of this, you can choose words, beliefs, intentions, and actions that help create the life you want."

This change of mindset means letting go of your story and any rigid thoughts and beliefs you have about both yourself and the world. These thoughts might connect to issues concerning trust, lack of confidence and self-worth, which are all underpinned by fear. You have to be willing to give up this investment in fear. Once you do this, life starts to flow.

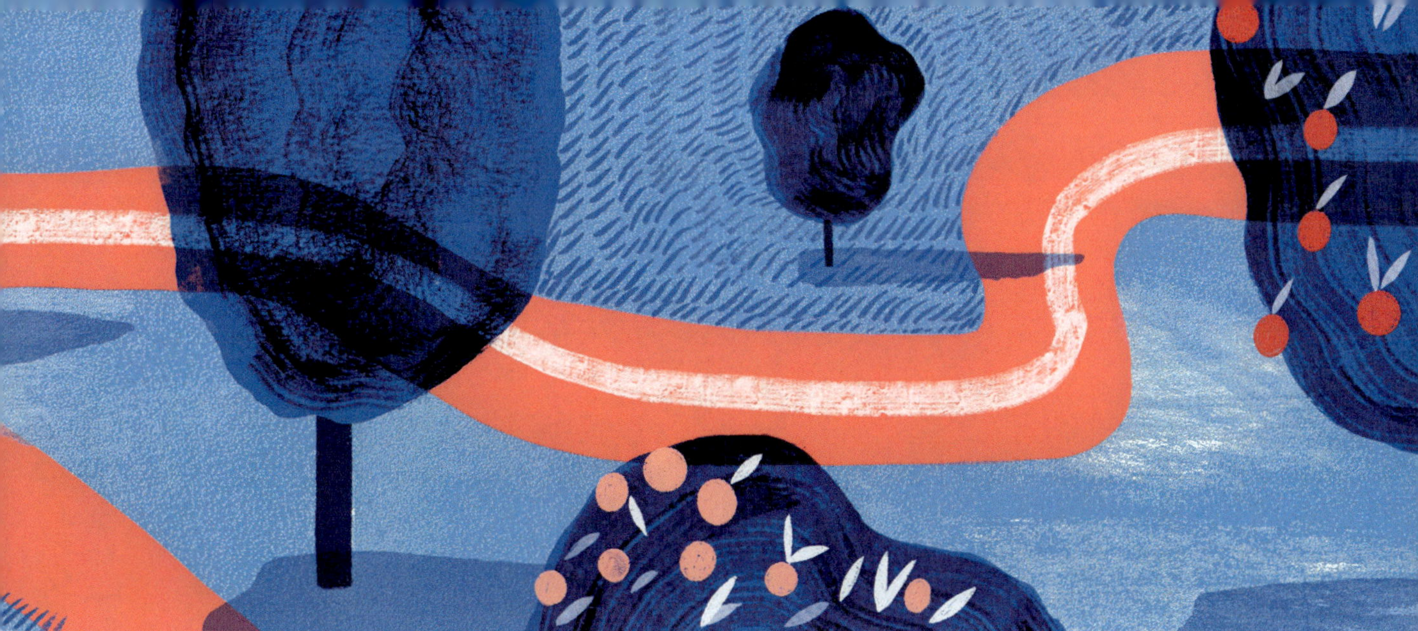

There are techniques that can overwrite your mind's current program to establish a mindset that is more nurturing and supportive and will help you move toward your dream life.

Puja suggests: "Start by writing a huge list full of all the things you want in your life. Nothing negative, no ifs or buts, just what you want. Then go through the list and actually be aware of the feelings and sensations you get in your body when you read a particular item. If you tense up, you're fearing that it'll never happen. If you feel smiley, it's likely that's exactly what you need to be doing with your life.

"Review that list and separate the items that made you feel tense. Those are the items that most require a shift in your mindset. By planning backward, so from the point where you're achieving that particular goal, you will soon see what you need to do in order to get there. Suddenly, the fear dissipates and the goal starts to become more realistic. Of course, you then need to carve out time to follow the plan."

As you begin creating a supportive mindset and moving toward your goals, be aware of tension creeping in. Stressing and overthinking can show up as resistance to change. When you feel this tightening sensation, focus on lightening up. Bring some humor and fun to the situation.

Puja says: "Be mindful of the words you use to describe your goals. Keep the tone positive and in a forward motion, so that you train your brain to accept the changes you're making to live your best life. If you believe that you can do it, you're more likely to achieve it because your will and motivation will always be directed toward that goal. Your goal becomes your purpose."

Changing your mindset so that you give up negative thoughts and habits in favor of a fresh outlook requires constant attention on a daily basis. But the effort is worthwhile. Through mindful attention, it's possible to get out of your own way and adopt a more optimistic mindset that, hopefully, will become your new default mode of being. From here, you'll feel lighter and more capable of moving toward a more contented life.

Steps to get you started

Try these exercises to change your outlook

What thoughts are holding you back?

Make a list of the thoughts, feelings, and beliefs that are self-limiting and keeping you stuck. Perhaps it's that you're not clever enough or don't have enough resources, or you feel worthless, with nothing to offer to the world. Dig deeper. Beyond these limiting thoughts, do you feel fear? Are you frightened that making changes will pull you out of your comfortable place and make you vulnerable? See what comes up for you, and then let it go.

Change your thoughts

For every self-limiting thought or belief, change the dialogue to something positive, expansive, and limitless. For example: "I'm capable, creative, and resourceful," "I'm worthy and open to receiving," or "I can do this." Truly feel the meaning of these words and invest in your self-belief.

Do three things today that move you toward the life you want

Intention is one thing. It needs to be followed by action. Susan Jeffers, author of *Feel the Fear and Do It Anyway*, says: "The only way to get rid of the fear of doing something is to go out and do it." So write down three things you can do today that will take you three steps closer to creating the life you truly want. Keep taking action every day, and do more of what lights you up.

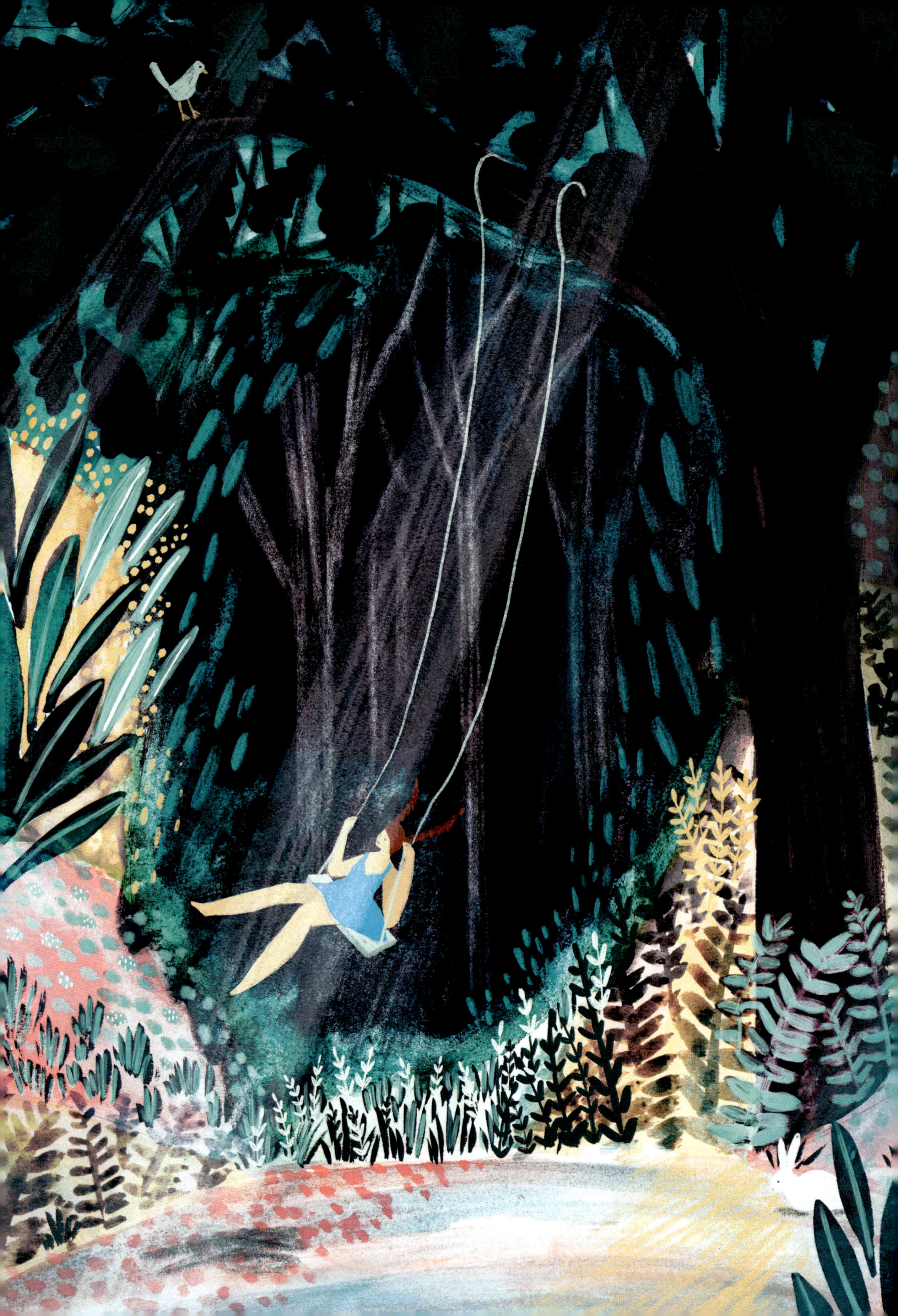

"You alone are enough. You have nothing to prove to anyone"

MAYA ANGELOU

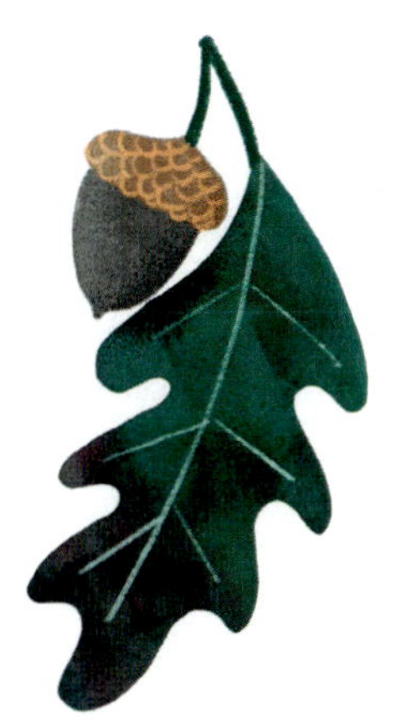

Let self-love blossom

Are you truly comfortable, confident, and happy in your own skin? Then why do you sometimes feel you should disguise your inner-contentment?

Self-expression is positively encouraged in toddlers, yet as you grow up you're often expected to "tone it down." Why is it that being totally comfortable in your own skin can make other people feel, well, uncomfortable?

Most professional and social settings, for instance, require compliance to an unspoken set of rules that generally forbid loud or overly confident behaviors. Often, when it can seem as if just being happy with oneself isn't "the done thing," daring to "love oneself" would surely result in disapprobation.

"Culturally, worth is attached to humility," explains counselor Katerina Georgiou. "Many of us have internalized the story of someone who contributes to the greater good over and above their own needs. Nurses who work hard for a low wage, for example, are the kind of people we've learned are worthy." Does this mean that everyone else is unworthy?

Conditions of worth

"I believe many people still struggle with the idea of individualism," adds Katerina. "When people just do their own thing, it can seem distasteful. Our culture has historically been community focused, and cultural changes evolve slowly."

Conflict can therefore exist between the desire to know, love, and express yourself, and the desire for external acceptance and approval. This is especially true if you've grown up believing it's not possible to experience these things at the same time.

"We learn what are known as conditions of worth in childhood," explains counselor Dan Tyler. "These are the conditions we had to meet in order to please parents or teachers, or any of the adults responsible for our care—in other words, we had to prove that we were worthy of this care. "Children internalize the values of whoever is the authority in their lives, and messages delivered in the classroom are particularly powerful, since this is where we're repeatedly told to behave a certain way."

If those conditions were to "be good," "not to make a show of yourself," or "not to make too much fuss" then that's what the child did to receive love and acceptance in return. Consequently, they may have learned that keeping a low profile kept them safe (as well as cared for). These childhood conditions of worth can form the basis of guiding principles in adulthood, which can feel confusing if there's a lack of congruence between who you were and who you are now. What's more, those who were raised not to make a show of themselves, could go on to be more likely to perceive self-love negatively.

Misunderstanding self-love

This might go some way to explaining why popular culture employs the word narcissism when describing anyone who seems too big for their boots. "When this term is used as an insult it implies that someone has no self-awareness—or that they assume an air of being better than everyone else," explains Katerina. Yet narcissism is a recognized personality disorder that involves excessive arrogance and need for admiration.

"Self-love and arrogance involve different behaviors, but we've somehow conflated the two," explains Katerina. "A narcissist's bravado hides what's really at their core since narcissism stems from a deep sense of shame. Self-love, however, stems from self-worth and the ability to look

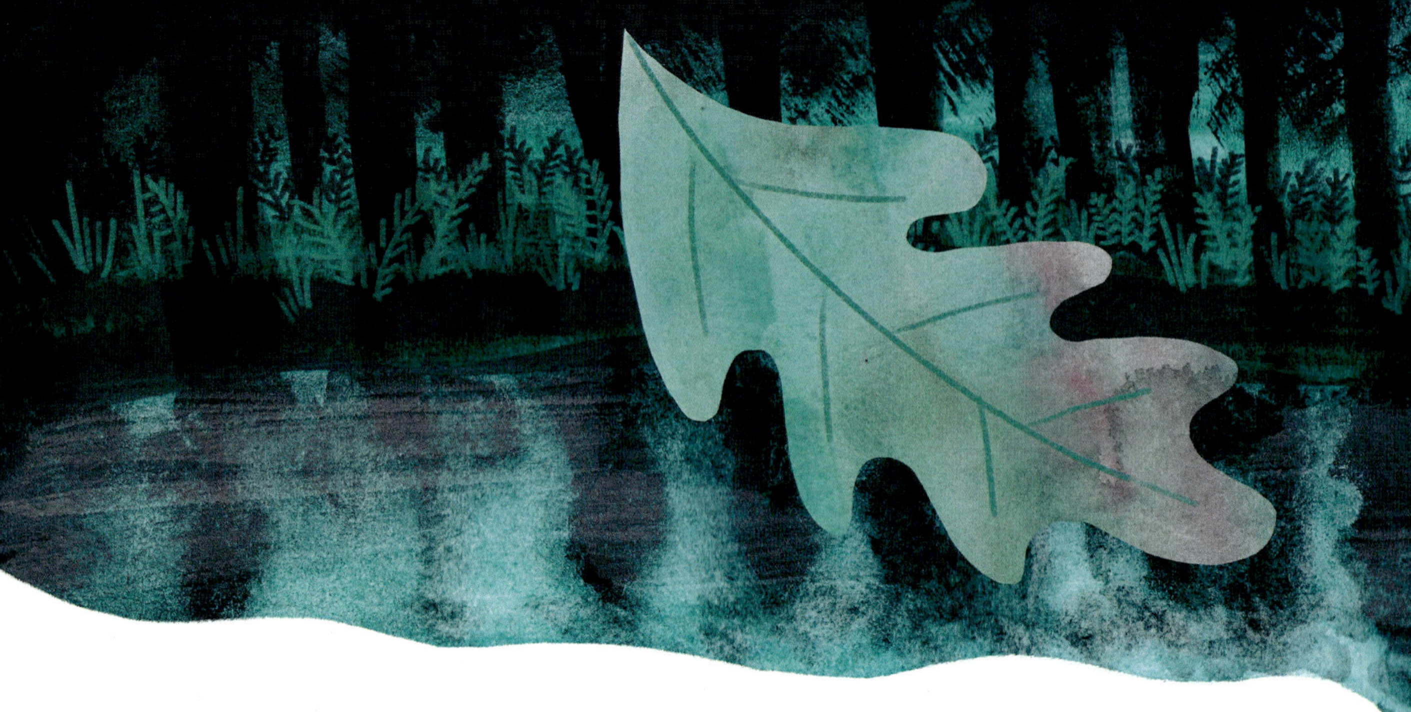

in the mirror and accept what's being reflected. "Besides, loving yourself is a nice thing to do. If a friend said they hated themselves, you wouldn't hesitate to help them in any way you could. So, why feel uncomfortable if the same friend 'loves themselves'? It's a paradox in society."

Overcoming the paradox

Understanding what it means to love yourself is key to resolving this conflict. Here, the acorn theory developed by the late psychologist, James Hillman, might help. He believed that each individual was born with a unique potential (like an acorn) that was waiting to be realized (and become an oak tree). This individual potential is also our personal contribution to the wider collective.

The acorn is essentially who you are on the inside before you internalize social and familial conditions of worth—so you might call it your inner-child instead. If you were able to reconnect with the hopes, dreams, and values of your inner-child you could also cultivate a deeper sense of self that's separate from the conditions of worth with which you grew up.

"It's possible at any age to experience inner-conflict between the values you've adopted from others and your own emerging values," explains counselor Dan. "If you once idolized a parent or teacher, but now no longer agree with their world view, this can create a sense of physical or emotional tension—but you can work with this tension. If you can identify which thoughts, values, or beliefs make you feel tense, you'll know that these are no longer true for you."

The good news is that your inner-child is always trying to be heard, even if you're not explicitly aware of any tension. "We call this 'directional tendency' in person-centered counseling and believe it's inherent," adds Dan. In other words, your acorn is always trying to become an oak tree, so why not give it a loving, helping hand?

Question automatic behaviors

If the seed of your true personality naturally strives toward growth and maturity, it doesn't matter if your life so far has been lived according to the rules and values of others. You now have an opportunity to keep watch for anything that no longer resonates. "Nobody is free from unconscious thoughts and actions," says Katerina. "Look out for those that happen automatically, and don't judge yourself for [having] them."

Question instead what you really mean when you say certain things—you may just be repeating what you learned to be "true" at a young age, so ask your inner-child why you chose to believe this in the first place. Do you still believe it? And does it serve you now? You can apply similar questioning to automatic behaviors—are you still trying to meet conditions of worth that are no longer relevant in your life?

Cultivate awareness

"Power comes when you know that you always have a choice," says Katerina. "You can keep doing and saying these things, or you can change them." If you choose not to change, and reject your acorn in the process, there will always be a part of you that isn't happy or fulfilled—and it's this neglected part of you that will reject people who 'love themselves' since they represent something unrealized in yourself.

"Ignoring this voice from within is like ignoring the need to eat," explains Katerina. "There's only so long you can go without food before it catches up on you. So, say what you want to say and do what you want to do, but know why you're saying and doing those things." Being aware is the first step step to doing something different, and daring to love yourself in the process isn't arrogant or wrong—in fact, it may just be the most natural thing you can do.

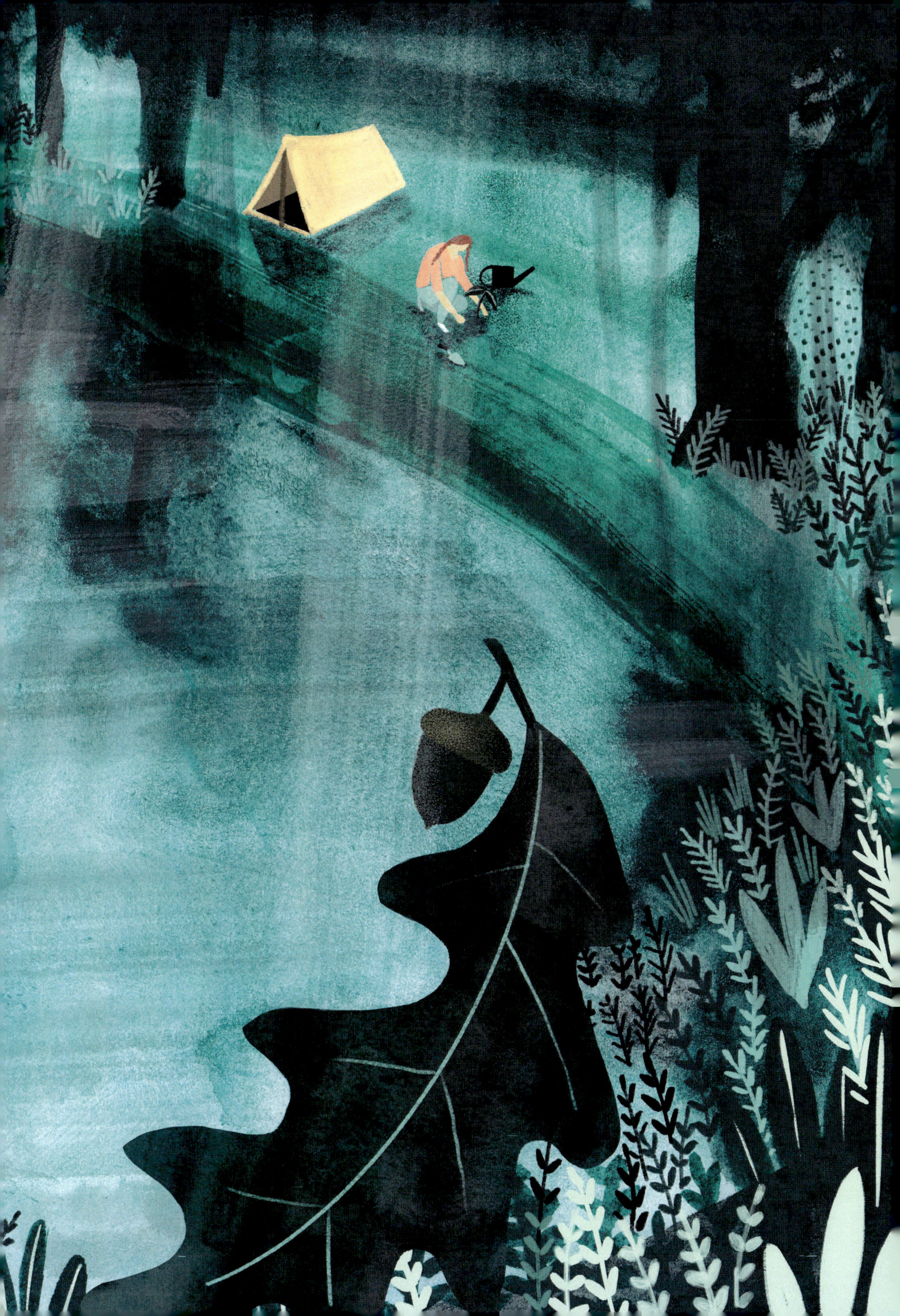

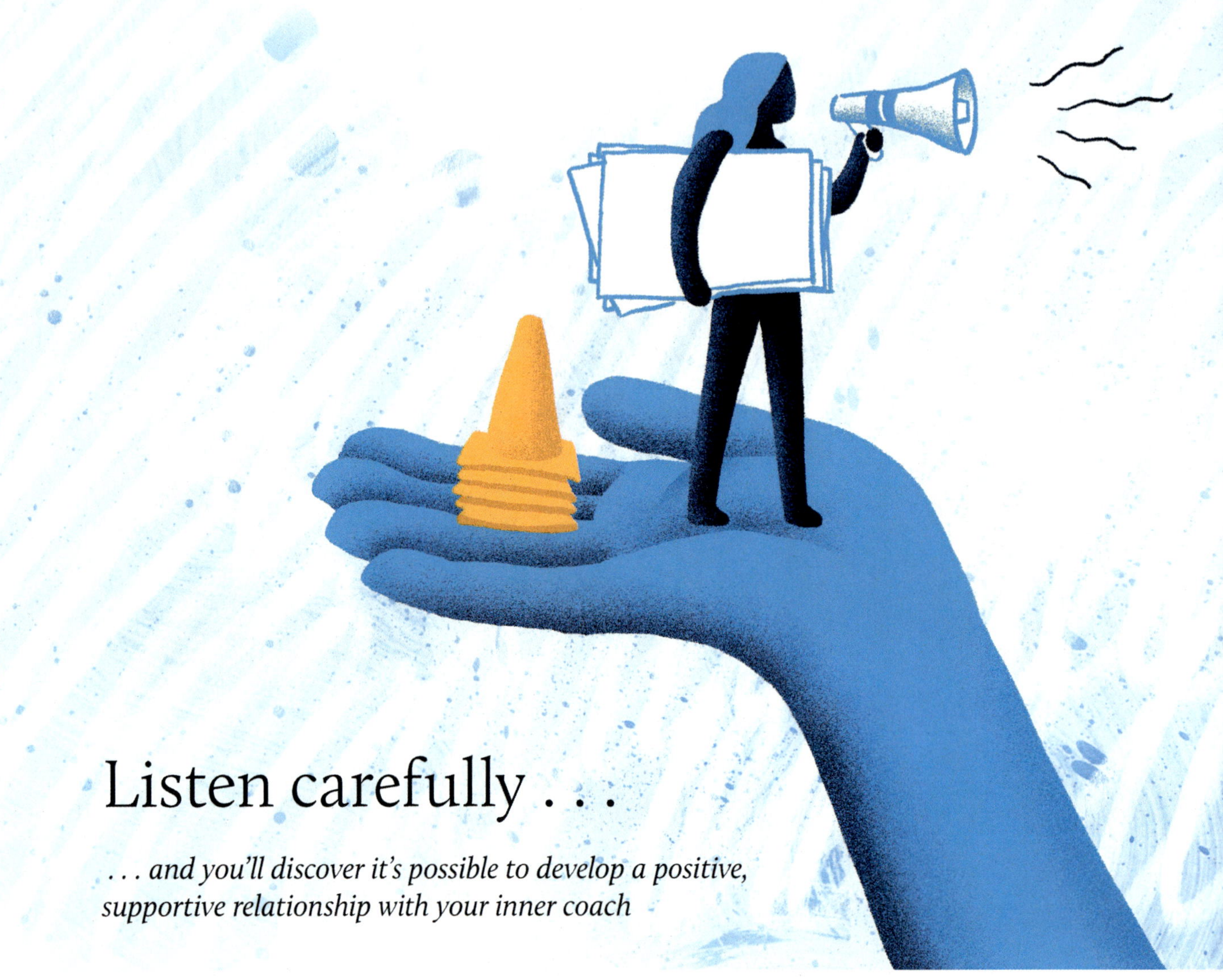

Listen carefully . . .

. . . and you'll discover it's possible to develop a positive, supportive relationship with your inner coach

Who are you listening to?

Imagine what it would be like if every day you could spend time with a supportive individual who wants only the best for you. Someone who understands your goals and plans and is prepared to ask challenging questions to keep you on track, someone who wants nothing more than to help you be successful in creating the life you want. "Sign me up now," you may be thinking. Actually, this is entirely possible. It's a question of getting in touch with and developing a relationship with your inner coach.

If you're pausing to think about this, you may already be able to hear an opinion forming. Yes, that one inside your head, your inner voice speaking to you. Perhaps it's agreeing it would be helpful to have such a person around. Or is it telling you they don't exist and, even if they did, why would they hang out with you? The inner voice is present throughout your entire life. It is often difficult to ignore and loves to share an opinion on just about everything, especially if it has anything to do with you.

Take a moment to consider your inner voice and how it talks to you. Is it kind and supportive, encouraging you to try new things and step out of your comfort zone? Or is it critical and judgmental, causing you to overthink, negatively influencing your actions, and getting in the way of your happiness? Are you actually listening to your inner coach or your inner critic?

The negativity bias

If you're in touch with and listening to your inner coach already—congratulations. Keep at it. You may, of course, sway between both voices depending on what day it is, what you're facing in life, and what mood you're in. But if your inner coach turns up more regularly, this relationship is going to be more positive.

Susan Ritchie, writer and executive coach and author of *Strategies for Being Brilliant, 21 Ways to be Happy, Confident, and Successful*, describes the inner critic voice as the "doom loop." She says: "It often shows up when you're under pressure and is the wrong voice to listen to at that time. It pulls you down. It's easy to get into a vicious circle of critical thinking and it can be difficult to lift yourself out of that mood." She adds: "We all have a negativity bias. This dates from way back and is a mechanism for keeping us safe from the predators at our door. This negativity is

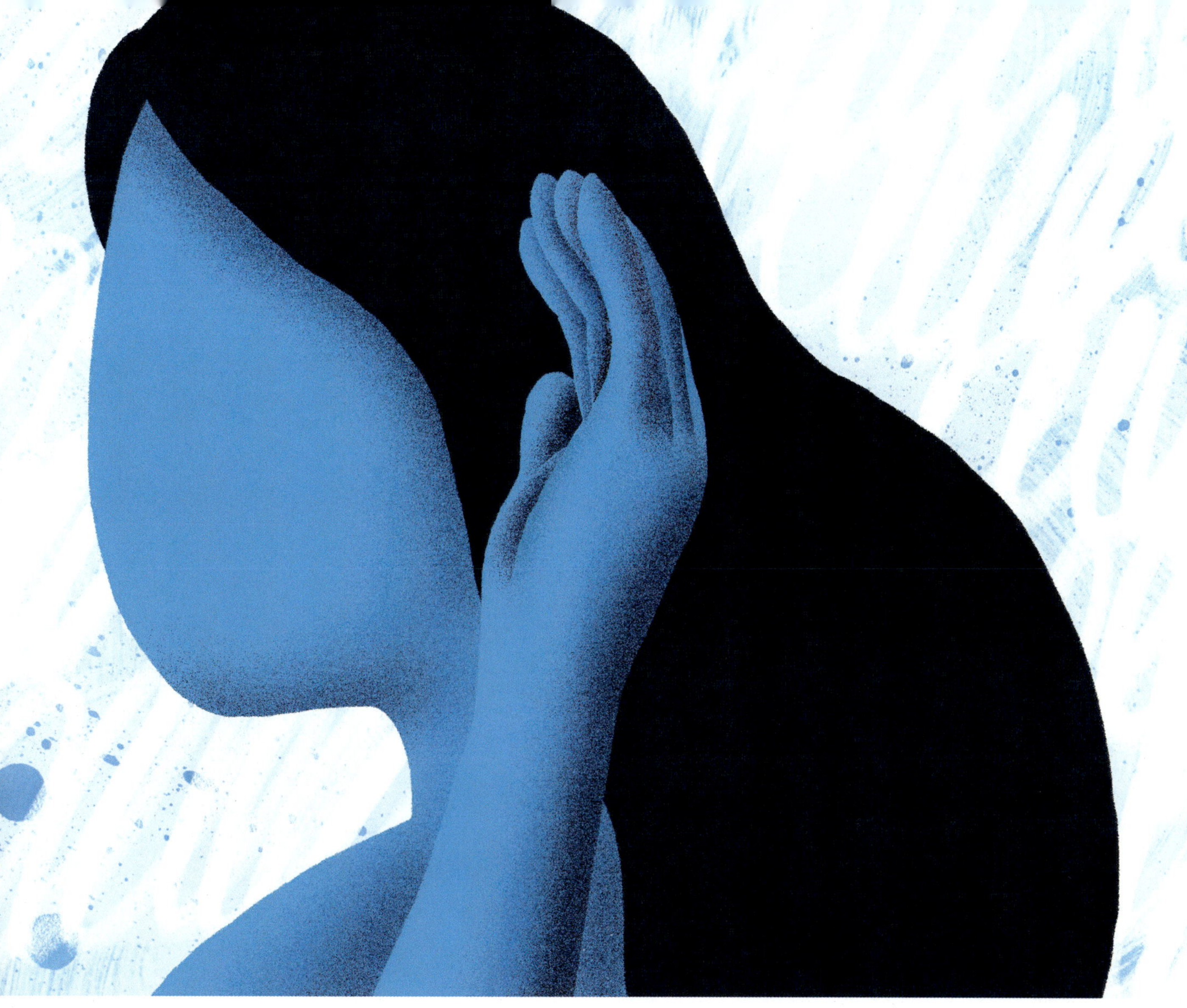

about surviving and is triggered particularly when we are under stress, a time when it's not the most helpful. We remember the more negative things."

It makes sense. Our early predecessors lived with constant threats and fear. Their key aim was survival and their focus would have been on receiving inner messages to alert them to danger and warning them to take appropriate action. In modern society and everyday life, it is rare to need the negativity bias for survival, yet the brain still functions this way, trying to warn of potential threats and holding onto negative memories and thoughts.

What's the alternative?

You've probably had the experience of doing something where four out of five things went well, yet you dwell on the one thing that didn't. Or perhaps a colleague or friend gives you some feedback—there are a lot of positives in it, but yet you still hold on to that one piece of information you felt was more critical. Rick Hanson, a psychologist and author, writes on his website: "that the brain is like Velcro for negative experiences, but Teflon for positive ones." So what can you do to strive for a more positive experience?

You might be thinking there's no escape from this critical voice. After all, it's inside your head. You can't switch it off instantly like switching off a show you're not enjoying on TV. One quick and easy way of lessening your critic's influence is to take away its power using some techniques from the world of neuro-linguistic programming. You can take control. Try turning down the volume so it's not so intrusive. Or speed the voice up so it becomes distorted. If you really want to have some fun, alter the voice and make it sound like a cartoon character. Surely you can't take those criticisms and judgments seriously now they're being put across in such a ridiculous way? These are instant methods of lessening the impact of the inner critic. Perhaps, however, you can nurture a more loving relationship and tune in and listen more regularly to your inner coach.

Why an inner coach?

Susan's work focuses on presence and personal impact. She believes it's beneficial to have an inner coach as "it's helpful to have strategies, tools, and techniques to help you show up in a more resourceful way and as a result be more

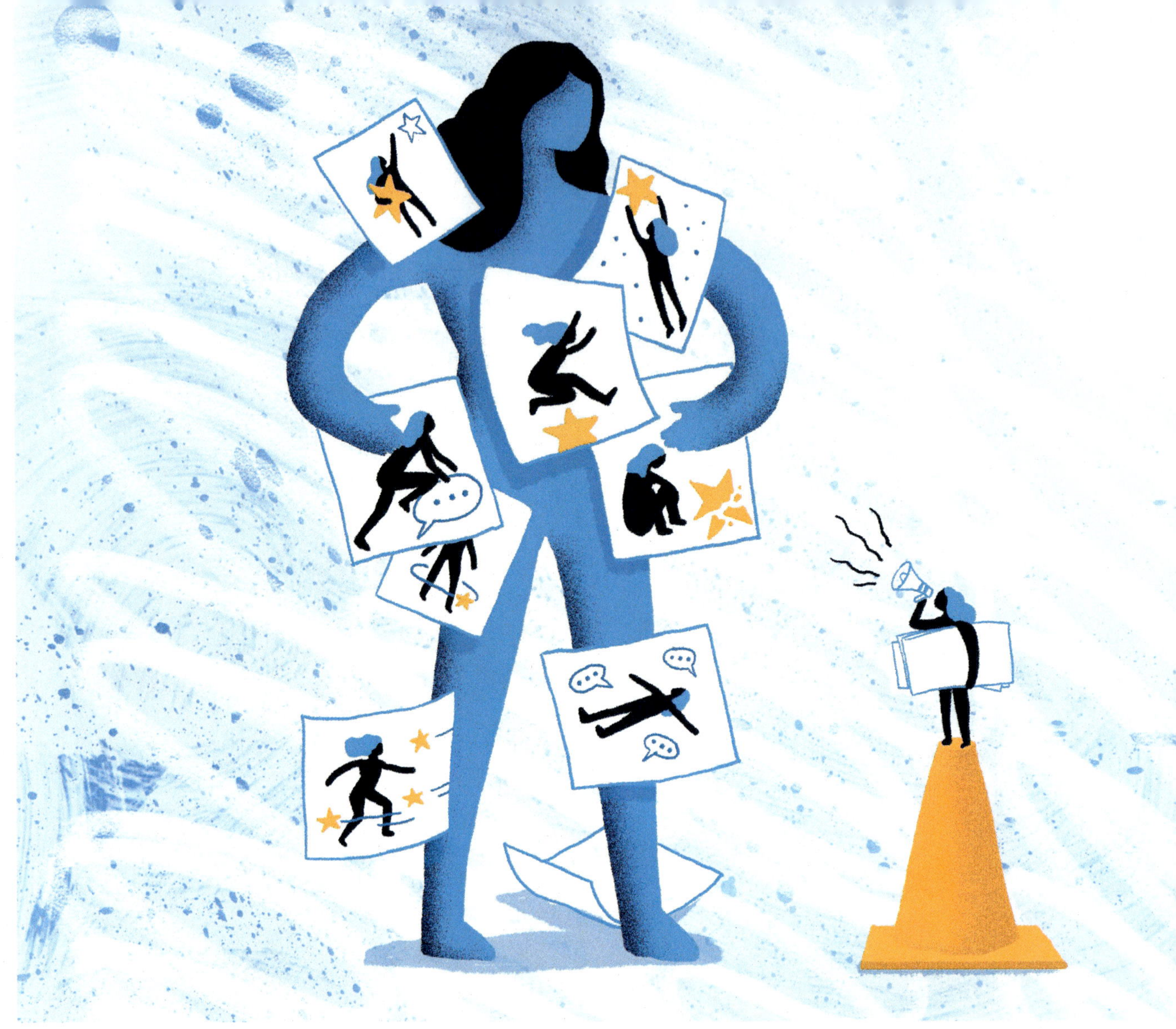

successful." She also believes it's useful to have resources that you can quickly tap into, especially if you find yourself in a stressful situation where you may revert to listening to that pesky criticism.

You've probably come across the concept of coaching. Athletes and sporting teams have a coach as well as many business leaders, and you may have friends who have seen a life coach. In sport, this person works with the individual to achieve the best athletic performance. You can't, for example, believe they would tell the athlete: "It's okay if you don't turn up for training today, take the day off."

Their role is to work with you to achieve the "best you." They want to support you to achieve your goals, often by providing positive challenges. They're not like your best friend who might let you get away with things. A coach will help you to consider other perspectives and weigh up the pros and cons of potential actions. If things don't go as planned, they'll evaluate the situation with you and explore what can be learned from the experience. And if things go well, they'll congratulate you.

A coach also has lots of support tools, which enable you to move forward to achieve your goals. Wouldn't it feel better to have someone helpful like this speaking inside your head? Someone who is there for you when you have a hard time, and encourages you to meet challenges head on?

Work from the inside

Inner confidence shows. You probably know someone who you believe has this within them—they undoubtedly face challenges in their life, too, yet they are resilient and go with the flow. In her book, Susan defines confidence in two ways. Inside confidence refers to self-worth, self-belief, and self-esteem. Outside confidence refers to the side you show others. She believes that when you get the inside part right, then outside confidence levels get a boost and you are given the chance to shine.

Your inner coach wants to work in partnership with you on all aspects of inside confidence. Positive self-talk, encouraging and supportive messages, and evaluating situations and experiences objectively are part of that. Try a few of the practical techniques (see right) to get connected and boost your confidence. If you want to be the "best you" and keep your inside confidence levels high, your inner coach is ready and waiting.

TIPS TO STAY CONNECTED WITH YOUR INNER COACH AND DEVELOP CONFIDENCE

Mind your language

Become aware of how you are talking to yourself and in what tone. If you detect mean comments or an unfriendly voice, think about how your inner coach would speak to you and rephrase the comment to reflect how they would put it across. Even changing a comment like "I should" to "I choose" can be effective.

Third-party perspective

It is common for the inner critic to turn up in particularly stressful times or situations. These can also be occasions when emotions run high. Your critic might turn up to create further drama. If you are finding it a challenge to connect with your coach or you want to lose some of the emotional attachment you feel toward something, executive coach Susan recommends "looking at broadening your thinking and changing your perspective." This can be achieved by taking a detached view. A good way to do this is to use a coaching technique known as third-party perspective, which helps you look at the situation in hand more objectively.

Think about people you know and respect and consider what they might do in this situation. How would they respond? It could be a family member or a friend or it could be a celebrity that you admire. For example, what would J.K. Rowling do or how would Oprah Winfrey react? Susan also likes the fact that "this technique can be done very quickly and in the moment."

Focus on the positive

There may be occasions when you've already predicted the outcome of a situation. You're worried about that presentation at work and in your head, you're nervous and flustered and can't remember what you wanted to say. Instead of focusing on a negative outcome, your inner coach would encourage you to focus on a positive one. Take that advice and visualize yourself presenting confidently, hear the words flowing from your mouth, see your audience smiling and enjoying your delivery. Hear the applause and register the questions showing people have enjoyed your presentation and understood it.

Circle of protection

If you are facing a particularly challenging situation, you may want to use a technique called the circle of protection. To activate your protective bubble, you envisage a circle around you or you can even pretend to draw one around yourself. Nothing can penetrate this line. It forms an invisible barrier that only you know is there and helps you to feel invincible. Again, this can be set up quickly—before you head into an important meeting, for example.

Ask open questions

If you get stuck on something and are not sure what to do next, work with your inner coach and ask lots of open questions. These are the ones you can't usually answer with a "yes" or "no" response. By answering these questions, you might find you come up with your next steps or are able to make a decision more easily.

Breathe

Don't forget to breathe. Whatever situation you are facing, Susan has one important piece of advice: "Breathe deep right down into your feet to help calm yourself down and enable you to a gain a better perspective."

BREATHE
YOU CAN DO it!
DON'T GIVE UP!
BE STILL and WAIT.

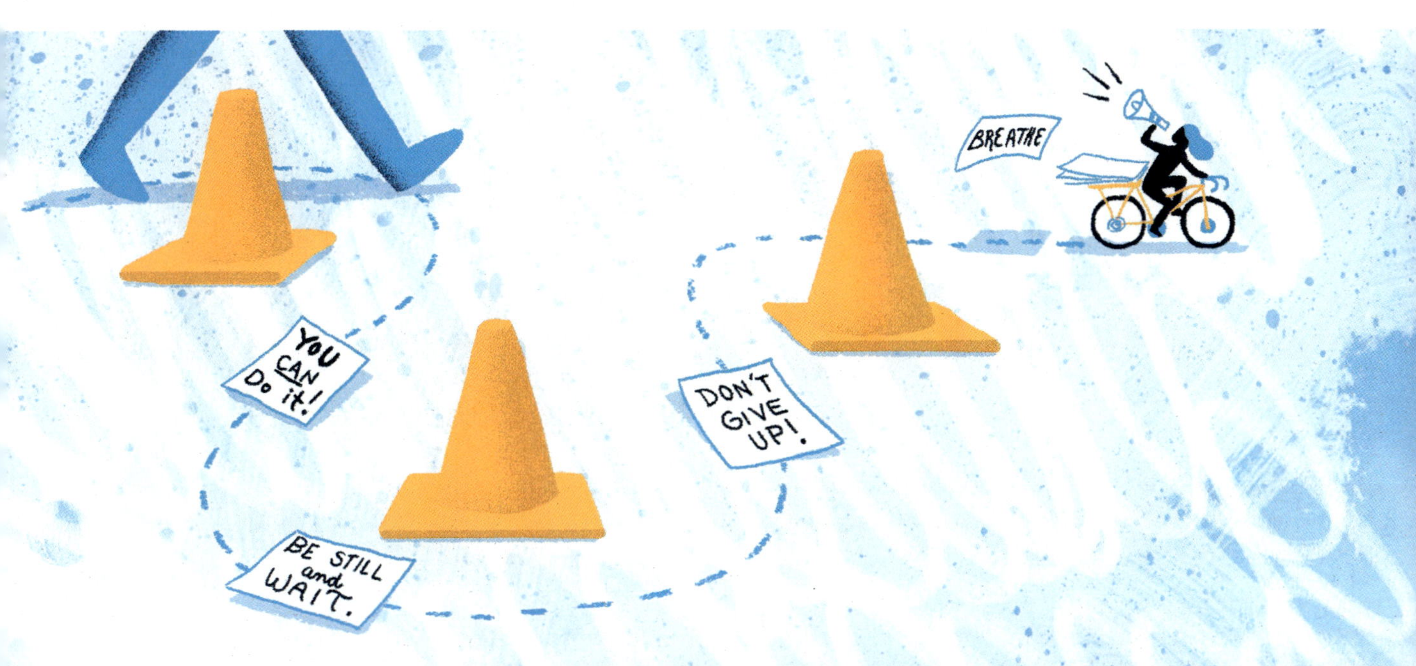

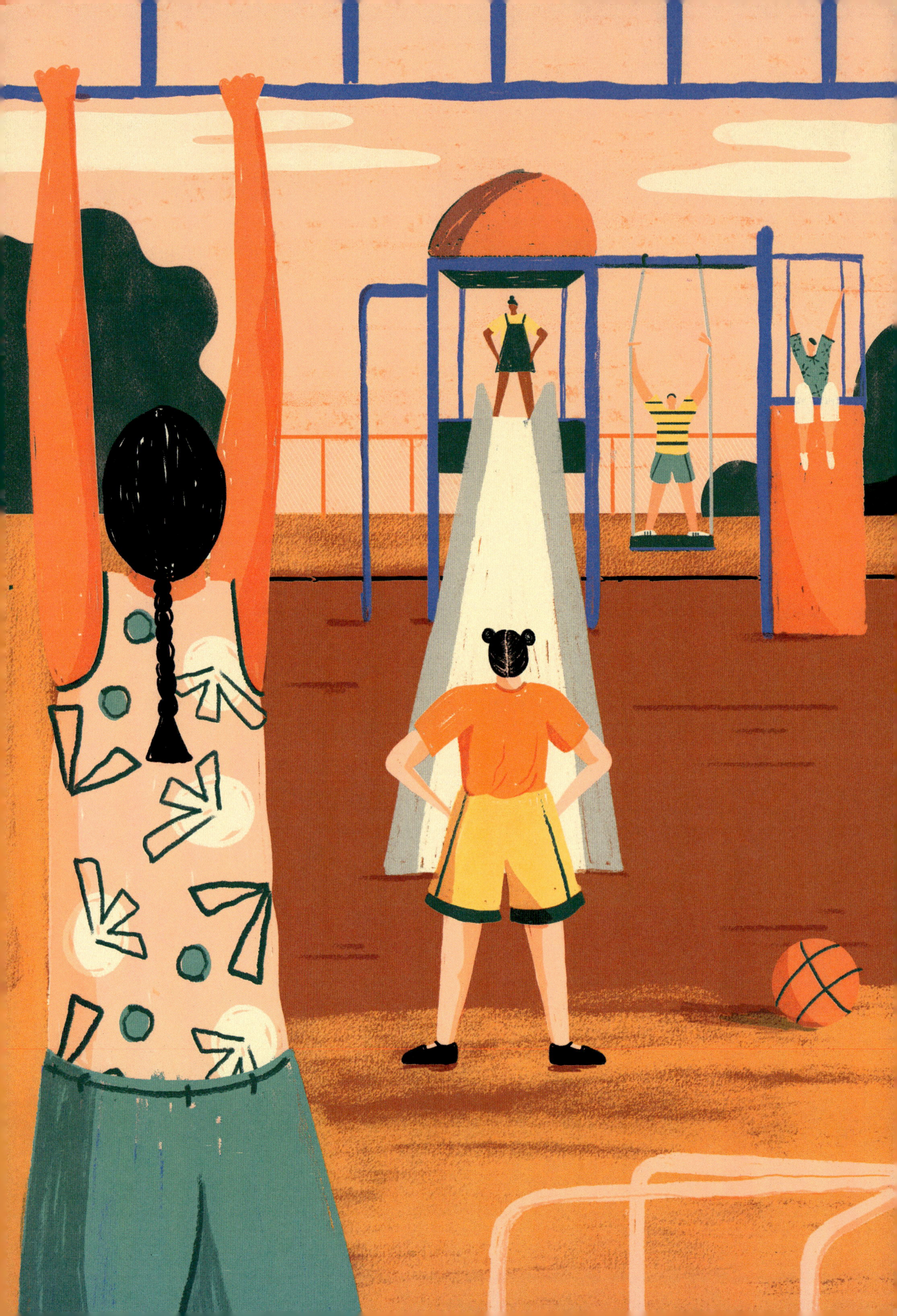

Make yourself heard

Do you ever feel that no one listens to a word you say or that your ideas are stolen by others? Here are a few ways to make it more likely that your voice will be listened to

Have you ever made a proposal in a meeting and thought it was dismissed, only for a colleague to put forward the same idea later on and it to be taken on enthusiastically by the rest of the team? Perhaps you felt a suggestion had been ignored by a friend, only for her to announce she's suddenly had a brilliant idea—exactly the suggestion you made two weeks earlier. Or maybe there have been situations when you've felt too nervous to voice your opinion, only for a more confident individual to say exactly what you were thinking and be praised for their insight or creativity?

If any of these scenarios resonate, you're not alone. Many people feel they're not listened to at times or wish they appeared more assertive to others. It's a feeling shared by Charlotte, 34, a freelance web designer. She joined a voluntary committee to organize events in the local community: "I made suggestions in meetings that seemed to be rejected by the rest of the team. A few months later, a colleague presented the same thoughts as his own and they were taken on board wholeheartedly. I wondered if I hadn't expressed myself clearly or whether others simply thought I wasn't worth listening to."

Why does nobody ever listen to me?

Being able to articulate your needs openly and clearly so others take on board what you're saying can be difficult. Nerves might stop you speaking up in a group. You might lack confidence in expressing your views for fear they'll be ridiculed or not taken seriously. You might worry about coming across as too aggressive or as a troublemaker for suggesting a less popular opinion. Maybe you're concerned others will misunderstand your intentions, that people will inadvertently feel criticized, or that your ideas aren't important enough. Or perhaps you do speak up but wonder why you bothered—nobody seems to hear what you're saying, you fear you haven't expressed yourself well enough, or your ideas seem disregarded as irrelevant or worthless.

Whatever the circumstances, feeling unable to voice your thoughts or believing others don't listen when you do, is frustrating. It can leave you anxious, lacking confidence, or feeling unvalued by others. But what's going on in these situations? It could be you feel you need to improve your assertiveness—a key communication skill that involves expressing your opinions clearly and openly, while respecting those of other people. Assertive individuals state their needs confidently and coherently and feel more able to make choices in line with their personal values. They're also less likely to feel undervalued or be on the receiving end of aggression. In group situations, assertive individuals are better able to resolve conflict and negotiate compromises that respect the opinions of all involved.

Other issues

It's important, however, to remember that communication is a two-way thing. There's always the possibility that other people really aren't listening, regardless of how assertive you are. They might not be paying attention, be preoccupied with their own thoughts, or be too focused on expressing their own views. In these situations, there may or may not be things you can do. In a work context, you could ensure your views are noted in the official minutes or follow up the meeting with a polite email summarizing concerns or ideas.

And what about situations when your idea appears to be dismissed, only to be suggested by somebody else and then taken up enthusiastically? Although there might be occasions when an individual is trying to steal your thunder, the likelihood is it's not intentional, but a natural side-effect of working in a team.

People often dislike the thought of new ideas and need to hear something several times before they can see the positives. You will have planted the seed of an idea with your initial suggestion. When somebody else expresses the same idea at a later date—perhaps having forgotten where it originated—others can appear more receptive. It's no longer a new idea but something they've heard before, less scary and something that, subconsciously, they've had time to get used to.

Whatever the situation or dynamics, however, there are assertiveness techniques that can help everyone to communicate thoughts and feelings firmly and directly. Learning how to place responses on the passive–assertive–aggressive spectrum can be a good place to start.

THE PASSIVE-ASSERTIVE-AGGRESSIVE SPECTRUM

People generally respond to others in one of three ways: passively, aggressively, or assertively

A passive response often involves saying or doing nothing. It can lack confidence and avoid the problem. People who respond passively might:

- Not say what they want or believe.
- Keep their thoughts and feelings to themselves.
- Go along with things they're uncomfortable with.
- Act as if they're not as important as other people.
- Feel guilty, helpless, or resentful.
- Have less self-respect.

At the other end of the spectrum are aggressive responses. These might involve anger, violence, and physical or verbal attacks. People who respond aggressively might:

- Interrupt and talk over others.
- Intimidate, threaten, dismiss, or insult.
- Undermine others.
- Believe their views are the most important ones.
- Not value, or even consider, the opinions of others.
- Try to control what others think, say or do.

On the midpoint of this scale are the more assertive responses. They involve expressing thoughts and feelings honestly and openly and respect all parties involved.

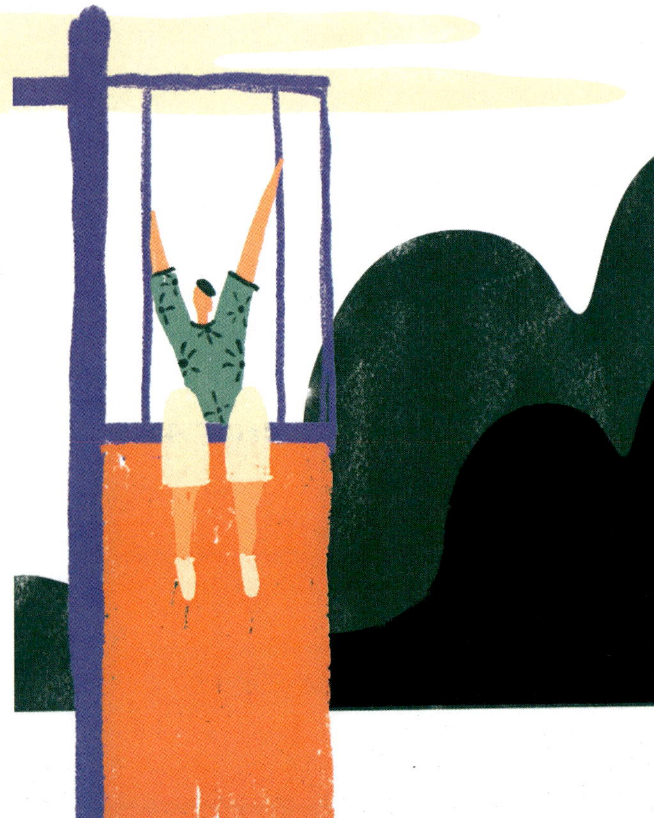

TIPS FOR DEVELOPING ASSERTIVENESS

Learning how to improve assertiveness can increase confidence in personal, social, and professional spheres

- It's oft-cited advice but body language really does make a difference to both how you feel and how you're perceived by others. Stand up tall to increase your confidence and try not to fidget—this can make you appear nervous.

- It might sound equally obvious but ensure you make appropriate eye-contact, both to show you're listening and to engage others in what you're saying. When nervous it can be tempting to look down to avoid the gaze of others.

- Keep calm and use a clear, steady voice. Be aware if you have any idiosyncrasies that could dilute your message—such as trailing off without finishing sentences or using redundant phrases like "if you know what I mean."

- Express your needs honestly and openly. Stick to the main points. Don't feel you have to justify your reasons or apologize for having an opinion. Remain polite but firm.

- Listen and consider the opinions of others even if you disagree. There may be some elements you can agree on or it could be that others are not expressing themselves clearly. By being open to ideas you might discover a solution that is even better than the one you were going to propose. Change your expectations from wanting to persuade others to think as you do to learning all you can about a situation and finding a solution that works for everyone.

- State your message clearly so others don't have to guess what you mean. It's easy for messages to be misinterpreted or ignored. What is it you want the other person to do or to know? "I'm planning on organizing a local arts festival" is a different message to "It would be good if there was an arts festival locally."

- Take responsibility for your feelings. If you feel angry or upset, remember that the other person did not choose for you to feel that way. They chose their behavior, you can choose your response.

- Accept that you can't change others. Some people you encounter might have poor listening skills or a hidden agenda. Remain polite and try not to take it personally.

- If you feel others are getting the recognition for your ideas, decide if there's anything you can do. The important thing might be just that the idea is taken up. In other situations, though, it can be sensible to put something down in writing.

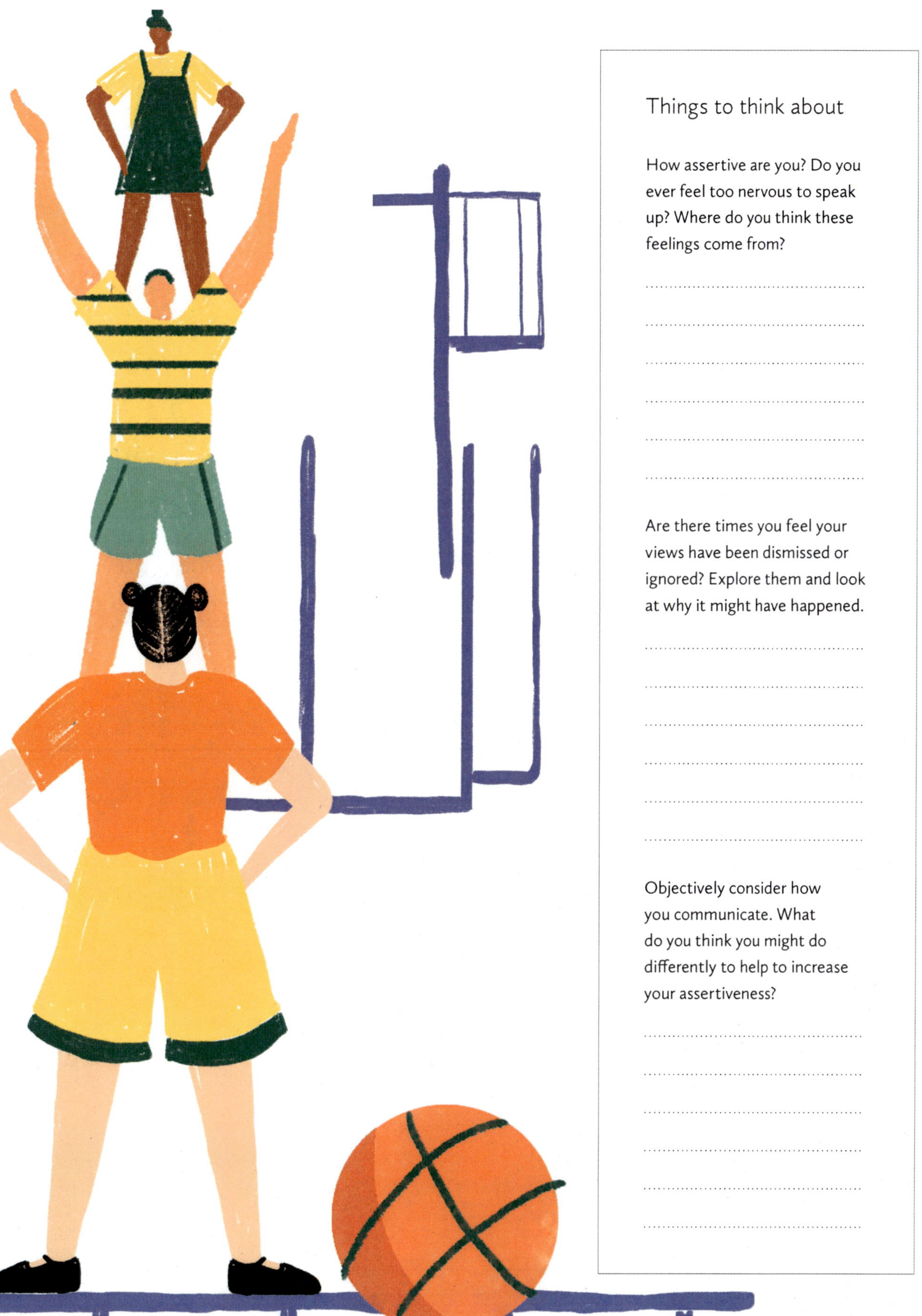

Things to think about

How assertive are you? Do you ever feel too nervous to speak up? Where do you think these feelings come from?

....

....

....

....

....

....

Are there times you feel your views have been dismissed or ignored? Explore them and look at why it might have happened.

....

....

....

....

....

....

Objectively consider how you communicate. What do you think you might do differently to help to increase your assertiveness?

....

....

....

....

....

....

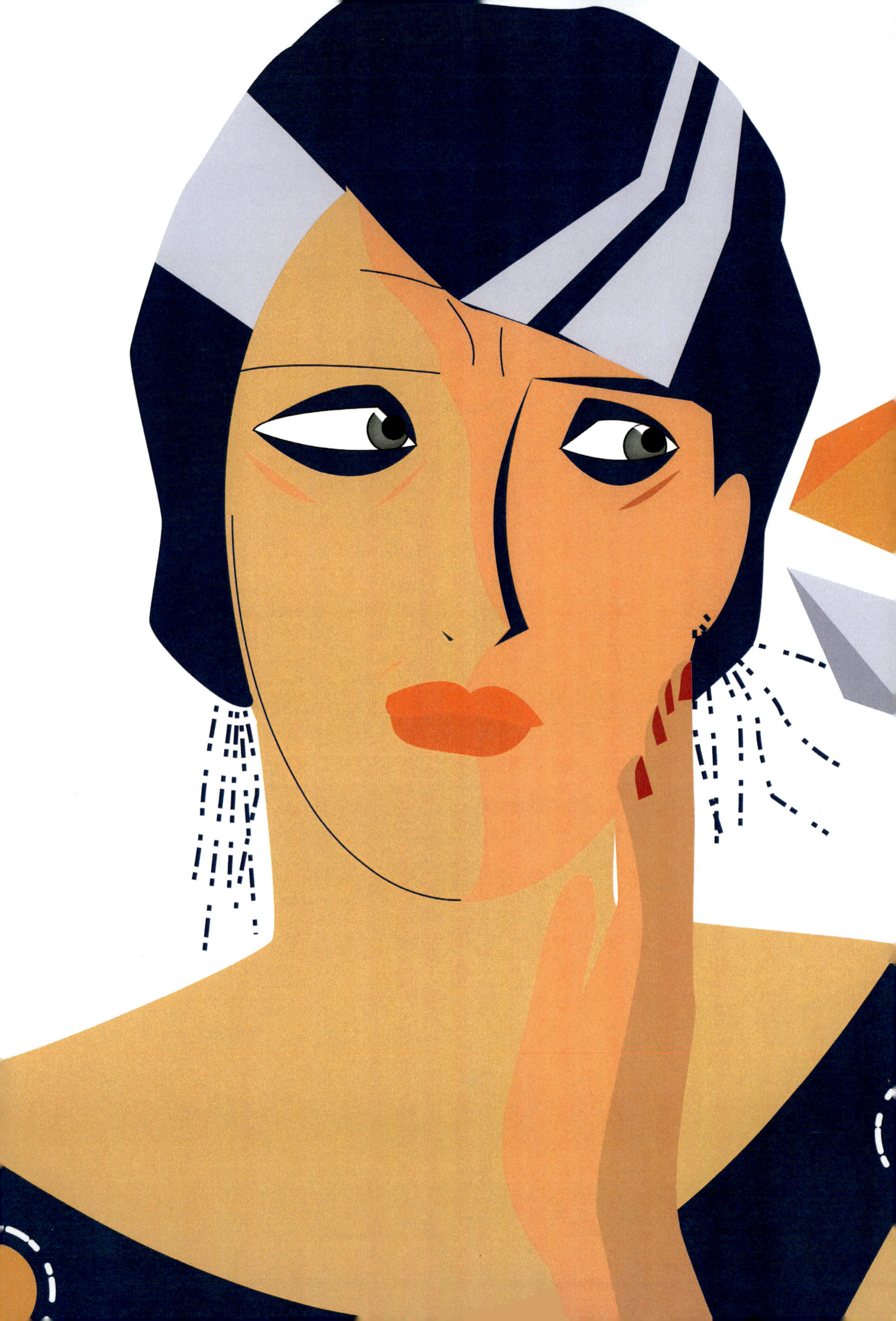

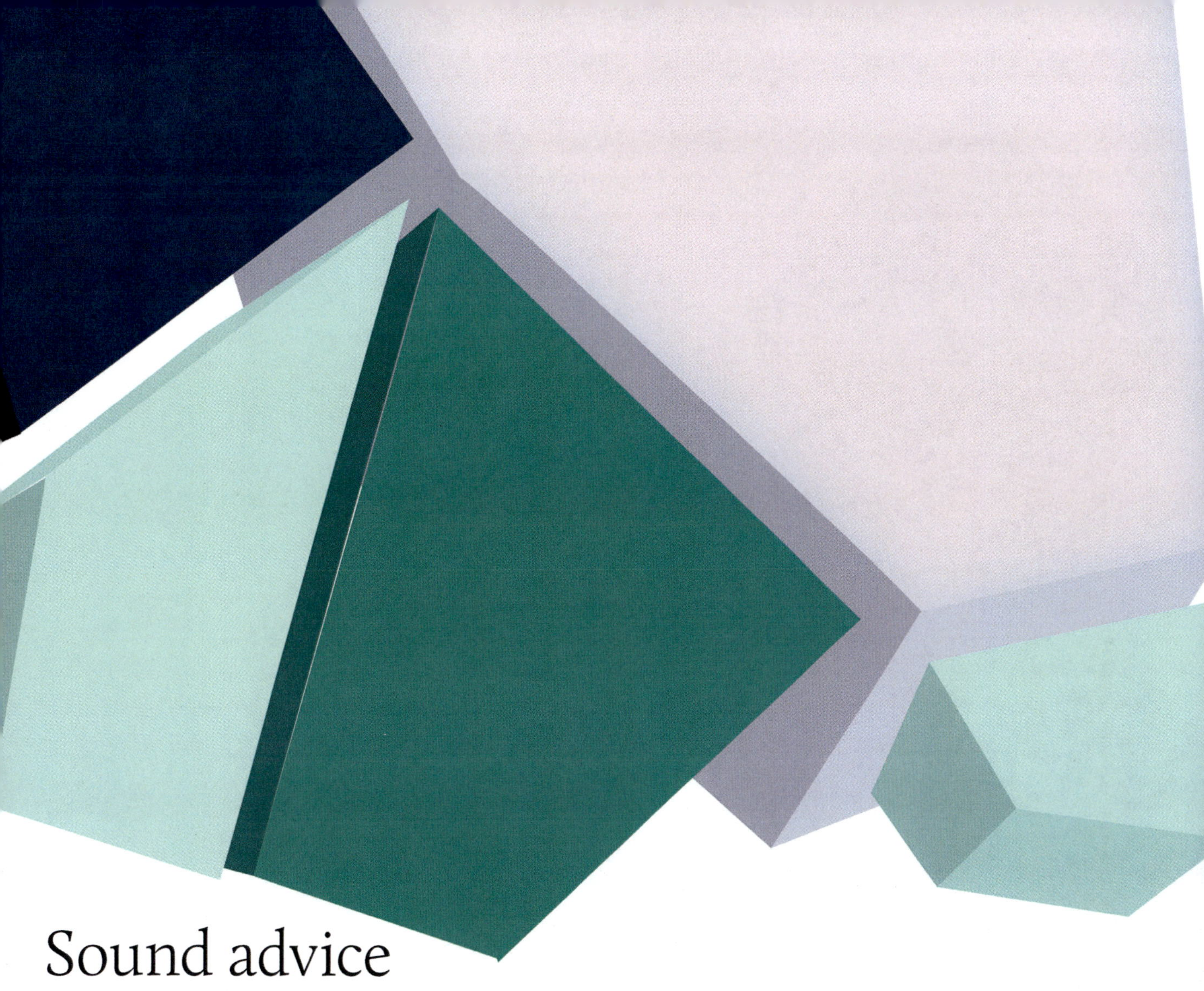

Sound advice

Regular appointments with the dentist and optometrist are the norm, but how often do you get your hearing checked? Few people do until there's an audible issue

Ears—how much do you value yours? In the league table of body parts, these appendages don't always receive the closest care and attention. And yet they play an important part in our well-being. Just think of the pleasure of listening to music or the radio, being able to hear friends and family—not to mention how important the ears are to our sense of balance, spatial awareness, and in connecting us to our surroundings.

I had a lesson in the importance of ears recently when I experienced severe problems with my own. It began with a pressurized sensation in one ear, which I tried to shift by joggling my earlobe, an effort that produced squelching noises deep inside my head. Poking inside my ear with a cotton swab would be stupid, I knew (although I was tempted). Unfortunately, it wasn't long before both my ears were blocked and my hearing was so bad that I had to ask people to repeat everything they said. Then I started to hear ringing and hissing inside my ears—and internal ear noise is no joke. When unexplainable noise is loud, constant, and close, and sleep and concentration destroyed, you feel driven to distraction. I suspected tinnitus and feared this would be my lot from now on.

With these types of symptoms, your physician is usually the first stop. But for various reasons, I found myself at Hearology, a firm of audiologists and ear, nose and throat (ENT) specialists in the UK. An audiologist diagnosed an ear infection and wax as the cause of my problems, and cleaned my ears with a technique called microsuction. The improvement was immediate, and after a follow-up appointment, a session with the company's ENT specialist, more cleaning, and antibiotic eardrops, my hearing returned to normal.

The experience left me with a renewed appreciation of the value of hearing and I decided to talk to Hearology's chief audiologist, Vincent Howard, about how best to look after it in the future. Vincent was 15 when he had his own lesson in the importance of audio care. He'd gone to see

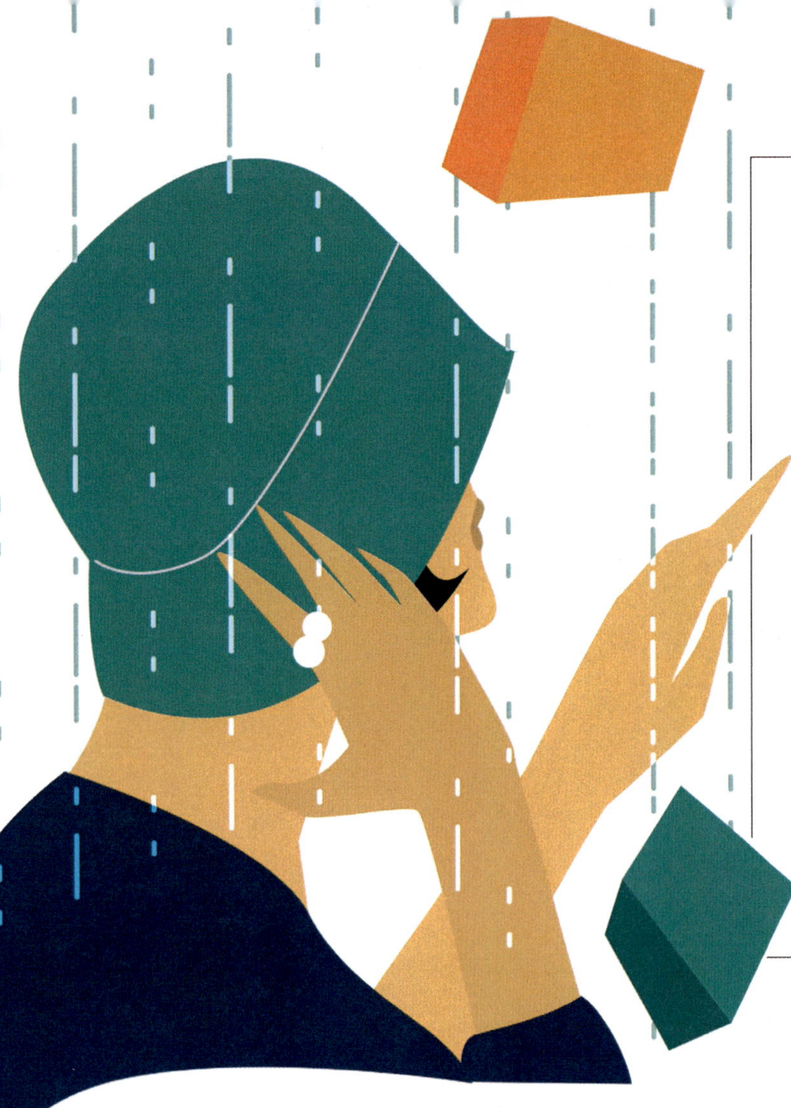

CATCH IT EARLY

It's time to see an ear-care specialist if you experience any of the following:

- Reduced hearing.
- Itchy ear.
- Recurrent dizziness/feeling off-balance.
- Constant ringing, buzzing, hissing, clicking, or roaring sound in your ear. This may be a buildup of wax, but it could also be a condition called tinnitus, in which case a specialist will be able to suggest individual and appropriate treatment.
- Sticky ear.
- Pain or an inability to release the pressure in your ear while on a flight or scuba diving.
- A blocked-up sensation.
- Discharge from your ear.
- A sensation of your ear being full or swollen.
- Prolonged pain in your ear.

Motörhead—once dubbed the loudest band on Earth—and was standing right next to the speakers when a head-splitting noise blasted out.

"I suffered acoustic shock, which really hurt my left ear," he says. "When I left the concert, I could tell that people were talking very loudly around me, but I could hardly hear them. All I could hear was a ringing tone." The ringing was later diagnosed as tinnitus—a doctor told him that the damage was permanent and he'd "just have to live with it." "The noise shock had eroded the tiny hair cells in the cochlea, which pick up frequencies in the ear," Vincent explains. "You can't repair sensory hearing loss, it's irreversible." It was devastating news for Vincent, but it set him on a path to learn all he could on the subject, and to study audiology.

Having become an audiologist, Vincent cofounded Hearology four years ago. He wants to encourage everyone to prioritize taking care of their ears. "Eye care has gone through an evolution in terms of surgical procedures. Teeth are prioritized from a young age—think of how many dental checkups you've had in your life. But how many hearing tests have you had? Maybe it's in single figures, or even none." He recommends having regular hearing checkups and tests, "so that you know what your good threshold is."

Thankfully, there's much we can do to protect our ears and hearing. Ear-wax removal is a common procedure in ear clinics. The wax itself, which is composed of skin cells, dust, and oil secretions from the sebaceous and ceruminous glands, is normal. It lubricates the ear canal and helps deter bacteria, regulates pH, traps dirt and dust, and repels insects and water. It also protects the eardrum. In most people, the ear self-cleans as we chew or talk, causing the skin in the ear canal to migrate outward, moving any wax with it.

But around 15 percent of people have excessive wax buildup for reasons that include narrow ear canals, more active ceruminous glands, or working in dusty, dirty places. Some also have a pH imbalance in the ear, which can be caused by shampoo that enters the ear and dries out the skin lining, causing wax to build up.

Syringing and irrigation, using water, is a common practice for wax removal. Vincent, however, prefers a technique called microsuction, which is a "dry" procedure that he insists is both gentle and directable. "Skilled microsuction practitioners can even remove wax that is attached to the ear drum and do so without causing any discomfort," he says. This is done with a tiny vacuum-like instrument, which has a surgical microscope that allows the audiologist to see inside the ear, including the upper part, known as the "attic."

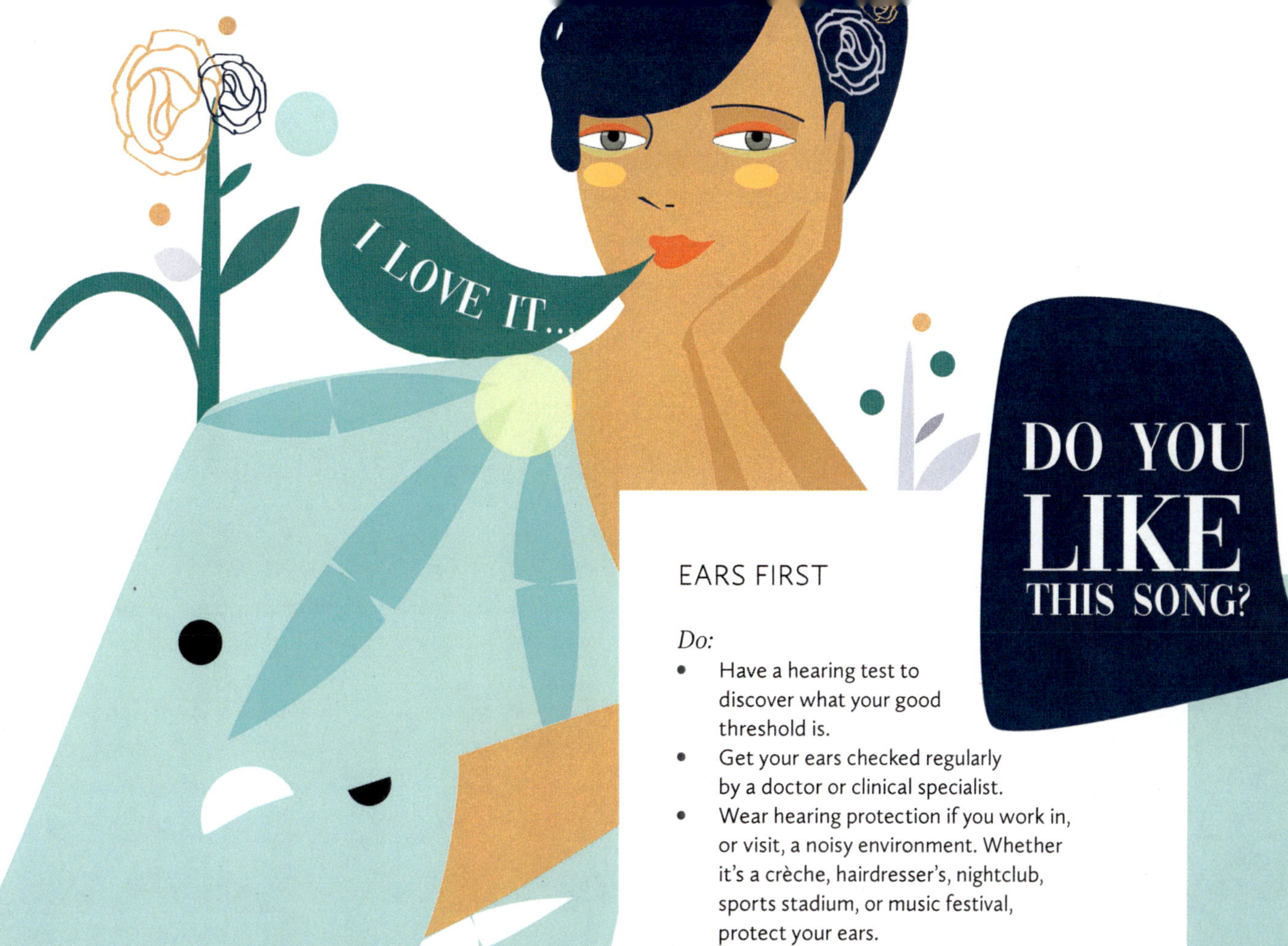

He also advises clients not to self-diagnose a wax buildup, or use olive oil or eardrops, before seeing a specialist, in case it exacerbates the problem.

There's also surfer's (or swimmer's) ear, where prolonged exposure to cold water or wind causes the bone of the ear canal to develop multiple bony growths, called exostoses. Over time, these can cause a partial or complete blockage, requiring medical attention. But shouldn't it be okay to get our ears wet?

"The ears are external, so it should be okay," says Vincent. "The problem is when the ears never dry out." For some people, water doesn't drain easily after showering or swimming. In this case, he recommends custom-made ear covers or swim plugs.

Hearing protection, such as earplugs, can help prevent tinnitus and hearing loss caused by exposure to excessive noise levels. Again, such protection works best if it's custom-made. For anyone who's been in a noisy environment, it's sensible to spend time in a quiet zone to "recover." Known as noise dieting, it's especially useful for musicians, nightclub staff, construction workers, and even people who work in a crèche.

Treasuring my hearing and looking after my ears is now a firm part of my self-care practice. And there's lots we can all do to keep them in good shape . . .

EARS FIRST

Do:

- Have a hearing test to discover what your good threshold is.
- Get your ears checked regularly by a doctor or clinical specialist.
- Wear hearing protection if you work in, or visit, a noisy environment. Whether it's a crèche, hairdresser's, nightclub, sports stadium, or music festival, protect your ears.
- Keep ears dry. Their reaction to water can be to secrete more wax to repel it. If water gets stuck in the ears, it can cause an infection.
- Avoid getting shampoo or soap in the ears as this can alter their pH and wash away oils.
- Understand what's loud—what are safe exposure levels?
- Keep earplugs and hearing aids clean.

Don't:

- Use drops or olive oil without first seeking qualified medical advice.
- Use ear candles at home.
- Poke anything into your ear—cotton swabs, a finger, car keys, anything. Ear canals have two bends and are very narrow, so whatever's in there will only be pushed in further.
- Put water into your ear. It will cause more wax to be secreted and, if water gets stuck behind wax, it could cause temporary hearing loss and create a breeding ground for infection.
- Ramp up the volume to block out all external sounds if wearing headphones to listen to music.

Garden within

Whether you want to grow a trailing succulent, some kitchen herbs, or a luscious leafy palm, now is the perfect time to get into indoor planting

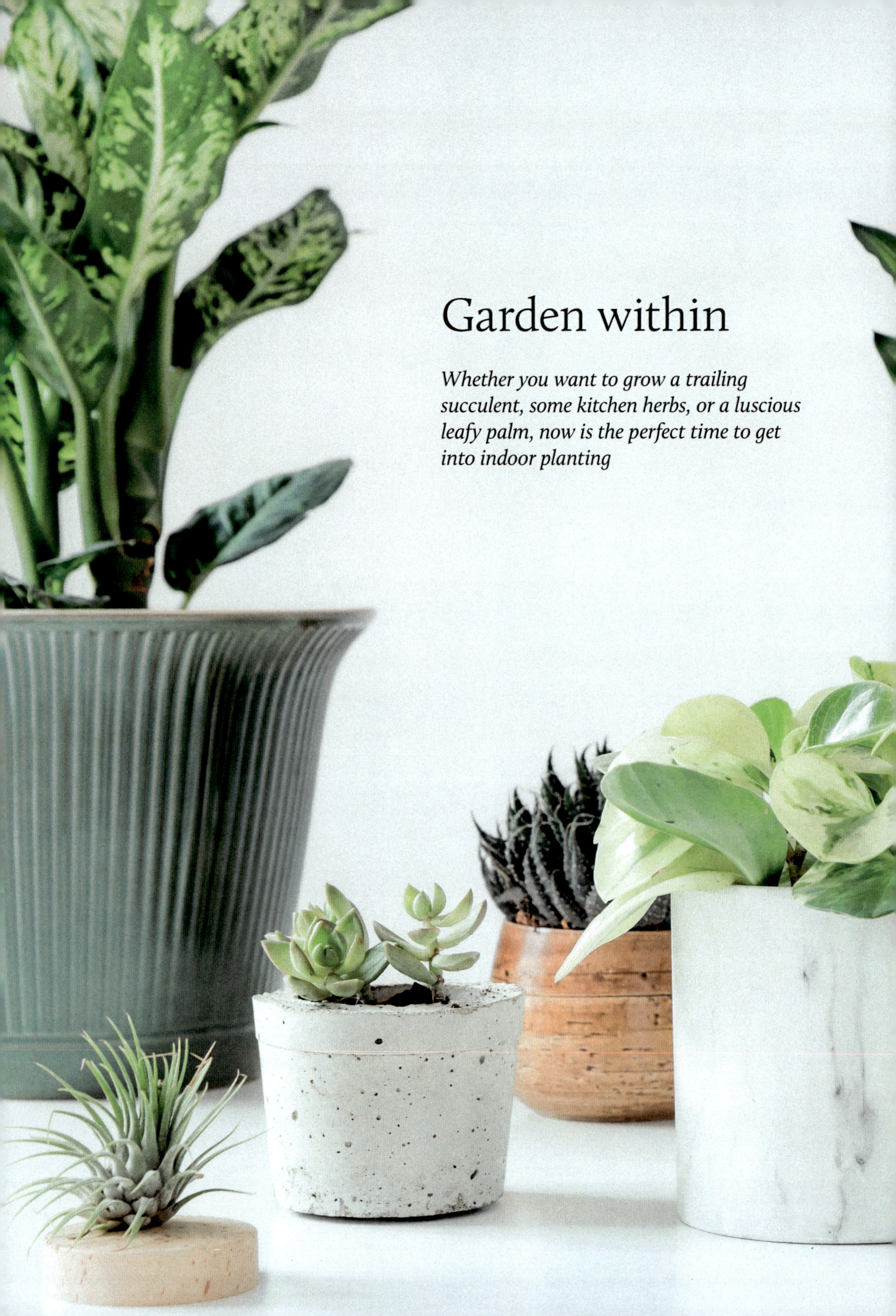

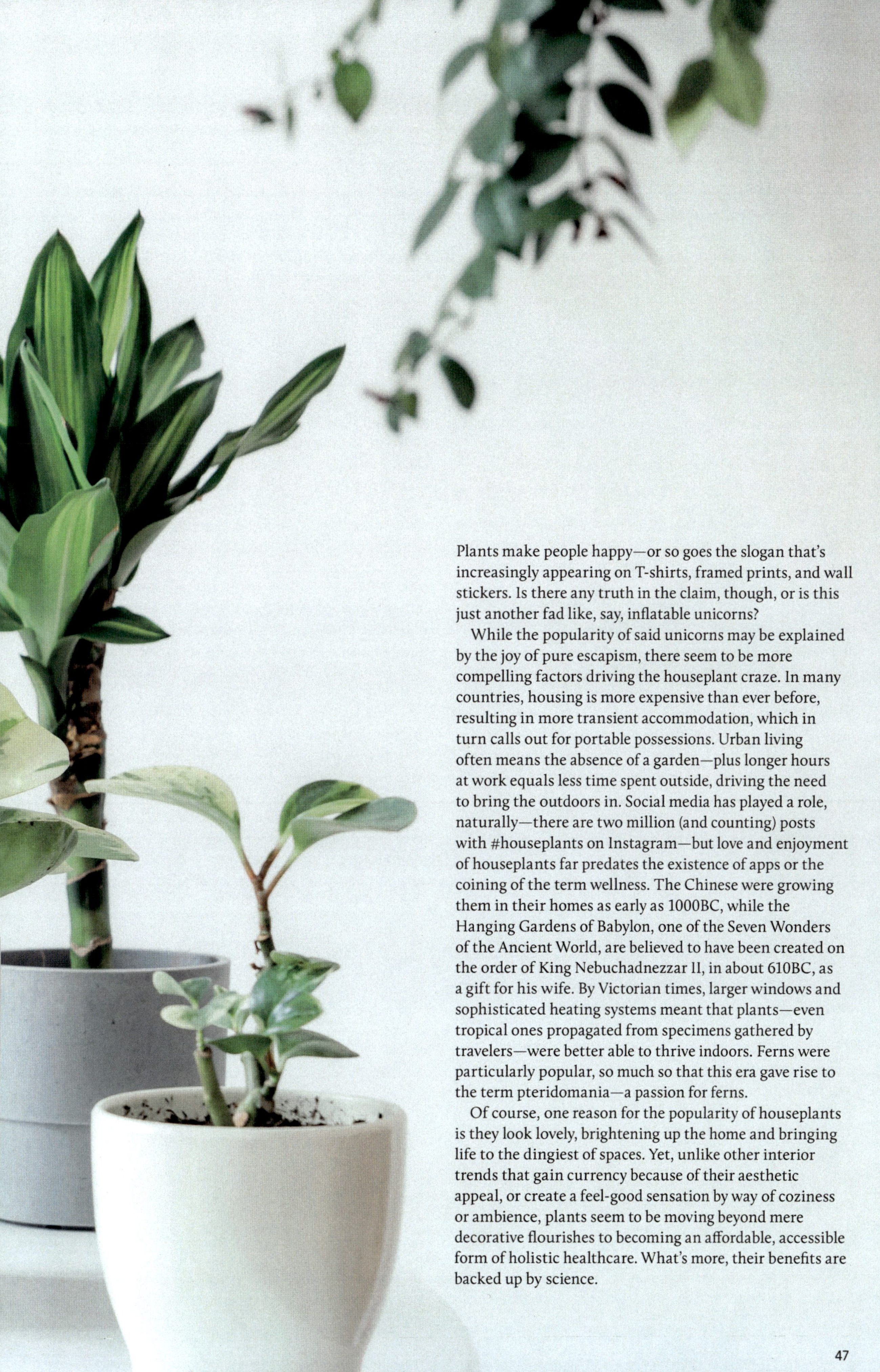

Plants make people happy—or so goes the slogan that's increasingly appearing on T-shirts, framed prints, and wall stickers. Is there any truth in the claim, though, or is this just another fad like, say, inflatable unicorns?

While the popularity of said unicorns may be explained by the joy of pure escapism, there seem to be more compelling factors driving the houseplant craze. In many countries, housing is more expensive than ever before, resulting in more transient accommodation, which in turn calls out for portable possessions. Urban living often means the absence of a garden—plus longer hours at work equals less time spent outside, driving the need to bring the outdoors in. Social media has played a role, naturally—there are two million (and counting) posts with #houseplants on Instagram—but love and enjoyment of houseplants far predates the existence of apps or the coining of the term wellness. The Chinese were growing them in their homes as early as 1000BC, while the Hanging Gardens of Babylon, one of the Seven Wonders of the Ancient World, are believed to have been created on the order of King Nebuchadnezzar II, in about 610BC, as a gift for his wife. By Victorian times, larger windows and sophisticated heating systems meant that plants—even tropical ones propagated from specimens gathered by travelers—were better able to thrive indoors. Ferns were particularly popular, so much so that this era gave rise to the term pteridomania—a passion for ferns.

Of course, one reason for the popularity of houseplants is they look lovely, brightening up the home and bringing life to the dingiest of spaces. Yet, unlike other interior trends that gain currency because of their aesthetic appeal, or create a feel-good sensation by way of coziness or ambience, plants seem to be moving beyond mere decorative flourishes to becoming an affordable, accessible form of holistic healthcare. What's more, their benefits are backed up by science.

REASONS TO GREEN UP YOUR INDOOR SPACES

Increase attention span

Research suggests that attention spans are getting shorter. Many people complain of their struggles to finish a book, which isn't surprising when you consider our brains are being conditioned to expect brevity by the short word-lengths of tweets, captions, and headlines. There is a wealth of information available at such a rapid-fire pace that it leaves our brains struggling under the weight of it all—something that was predicted by Nobel Prize-winning economist Herbert Simon back in 1977, when he cautioned that information consumes "the attention of its recipients. Hence a wealth of information creates a poverty of attention." Fortunately, according to a study published in the *Journal of Environmental Psychology*, plants have a positive impact on improving concentration. So if Leo Tolstoy's *War and Peace* is on this year's reading agenda, filling the home with living specimens could help increase the attention span required for the task. These findings bear relevance to workspaces, too—a 2014 study found that enriching relatively bare offices with plants increased productivity by 15 percent.

Aid recovery

It's common to give flowers to someone who's unwell, or recovering from illness, but research suggests a potted plant could be an even better option. A study published in *Science Daily* revealed patients with plants in their rooms required significantly less medication for pain, recuperated more quickly, and demonstrated positive physiological responses, such as lower blood pressure and heart rate. This suggests that plants have medicinal qualities, regardless of whether they're ground to a paste or steeped in boiling water, which often happens in traditional remedies.

Clean the air

Even before the current pandemic, World Health Organization research demonstrated that humans were spending more time indoors than ever before. In some countries, it's estimated that people spend 90 percent of their lives inside. Unfortunately, indoor settings are increasingly filled with toxins from cleaning liquids and sprays, plus decorating and grooming products, as well as emissions from gas- and wood-burners. Something as seemingly innocuous as drying laundry indoors can add to the problem, as does, of course, poor ventilation. A Clean Air Study, conducted by NASA, found that houseplants absorbed common household toxins and purified the air, making breathing safer and easier.

Spark creativity

Many people have probably experienced that blanket of nothingness that sometimes settles over the mind, the mental block that makes it difficult to think or create—yet creativity, or having an outlet in which to make and do, is known to be good for the soul. The good news is that, according to research conducted by Texas A&M University, having plants around can boost creativity and enhance the ability to come up with ideas, which might help alleviate feelings of anxiety.

Boost empathy

Perhaps it's the mere fact of giving something care, and experiencing the pleasure of watching it grow, but it's been suggested that even minimal interaction with plants can make people kinder and more empathetic. Experiments carried out at the University of California, Berkeley, saw participants filling out unrelated questionnaires while seated at tables on which a greater or fewer numbers of plants were placed. At the end of this dummy session, they were told they were free to leave, but that they could also, if they wanted, stay and make paper cranes for a Japanese relief-effort program. There was a direct link between the number of cranes made and the presence of plants, leading researchers to conclude they boost positive emotions and, consequently, positive behaviors.

Encourage sleep

Most people have experienced the discomfort that comes with missed sleep, whether from a disturbed night, or from short- or long-term insomnia. Elevated cortisol levels have been seen to play a role in disrupted sleep, so it's interesting to note that plants could be useful in reducing them. Those that release oxygen, rather than carbon dioxide, are best here, so choose varieties like jasmine, valerian, lavender, aloe vera, and snake plant for the bedroom.

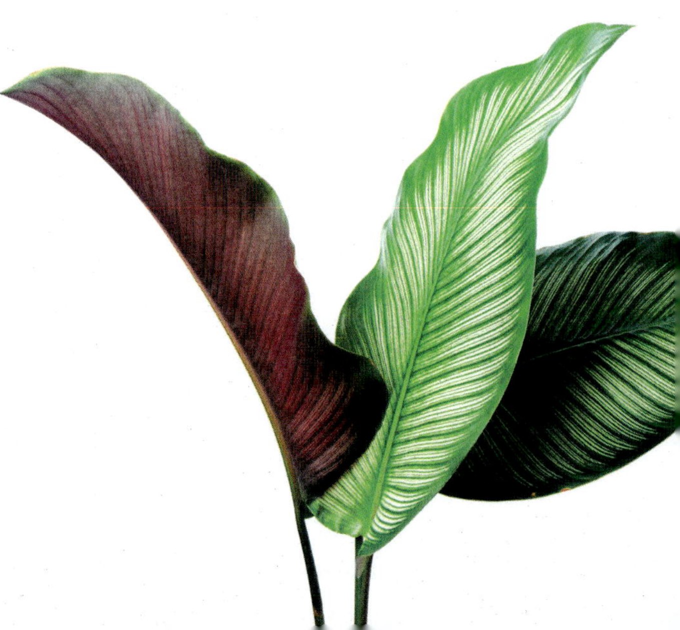

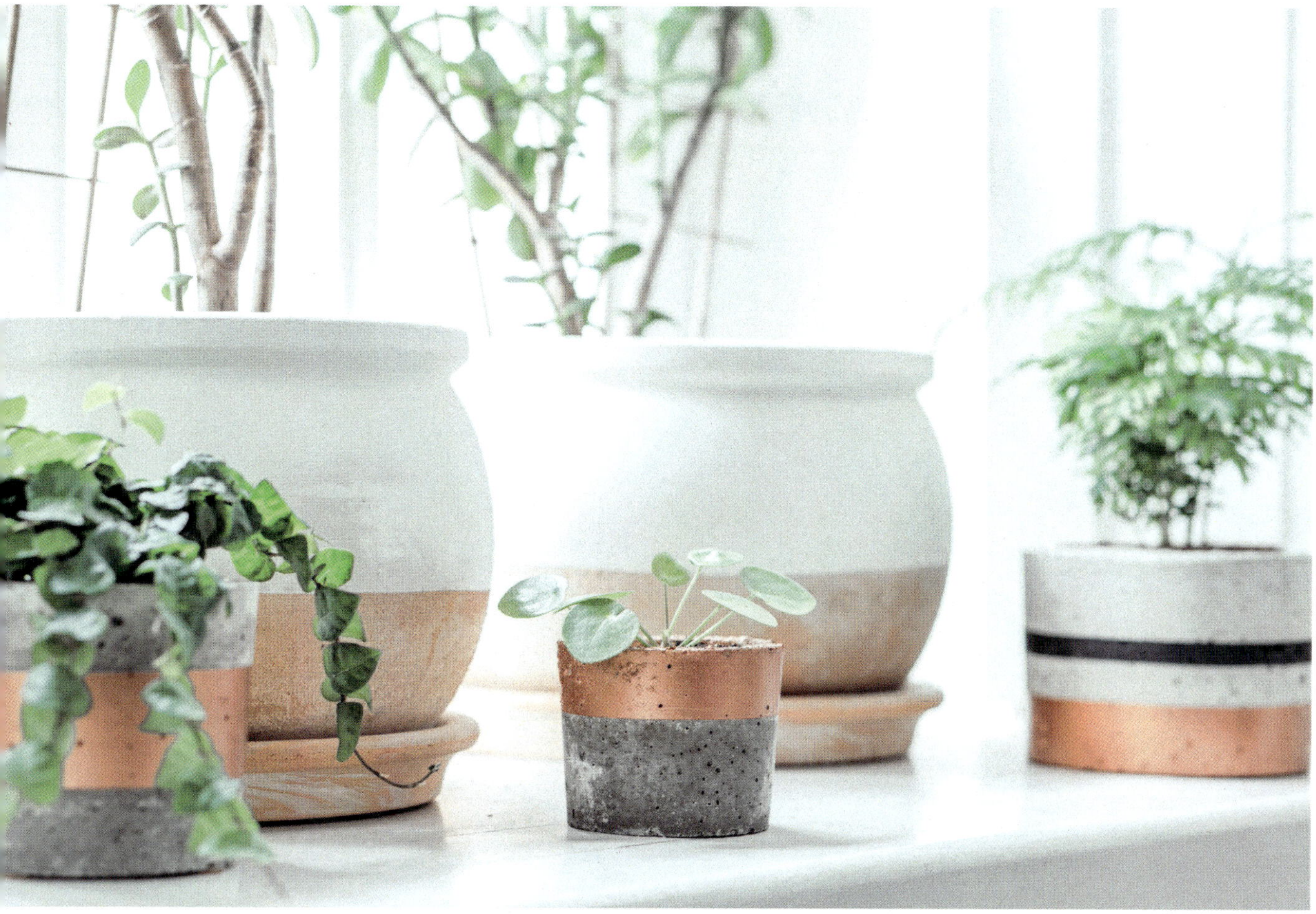

BEST HOUSEPLANTS FOR . . .

Beginners

The spider plant, with its long, variegated leaves, grows easily and quickly, making it a good choice (and encouragingly fulfilling) for the plant novice. The wispy plantlets that they shoot out from their longest stems are incredibly satisfying to witness and can be replanted to make new plants. They can withstand all kinds of water, light, and temperature levels, so are ideal for the plant-nervous individual.

Sleep

The comforting scent of jasmine has long been known to encourage and enhance sleep, but it doesn't need to be experienced by way of aromatherapy oils. Those starry flowers, placed next to the bed, will boost relaxation by way of their scent, adding another layer of comfort on top of that provided by the plant's stress-busting greenery.

Air quality

Rubber plants not only look impressive, with their sturdy, glossy leaves, but they're also adept at sucking up harmful toxins. NASA-funded research back in 1989, which investigated the best plants for air filtration, also suggests chrysanthemum, gerbera daisies, and English ivy.

Anxiety

Nicknamed mother-in-law's tongue, the snake plant is actually one of the best choices for reducing anxious feelings. It's also thought that it might help ease headaches and boost concentration and energy levels.

Pets

Not all houseplants are created equal and sadly some (such as aloe vera, sago palm, and weeping fig) can be toxic to furry friends. Since cats and dogs are also known stress relievers, it would be a shame to jeopardize one with the existence of the other. The money tree is not only effective at removing toxins from the air but is also believed by some to enhance prosperity. Best of all, it's completely pet-friendly.

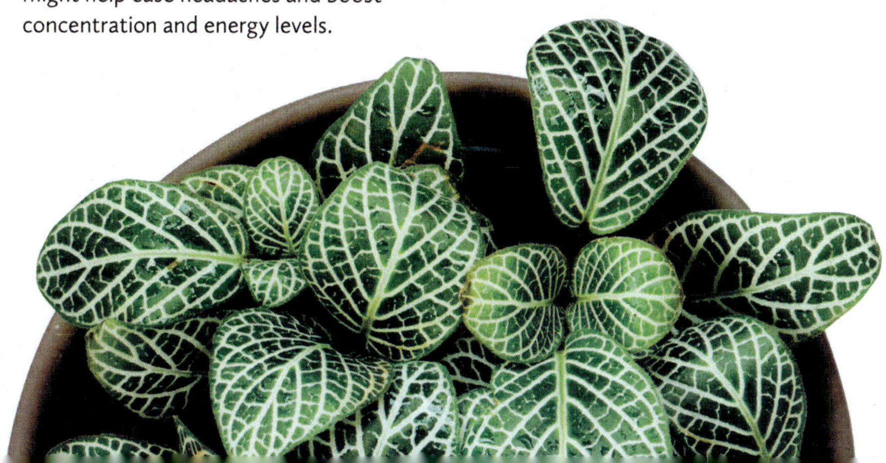

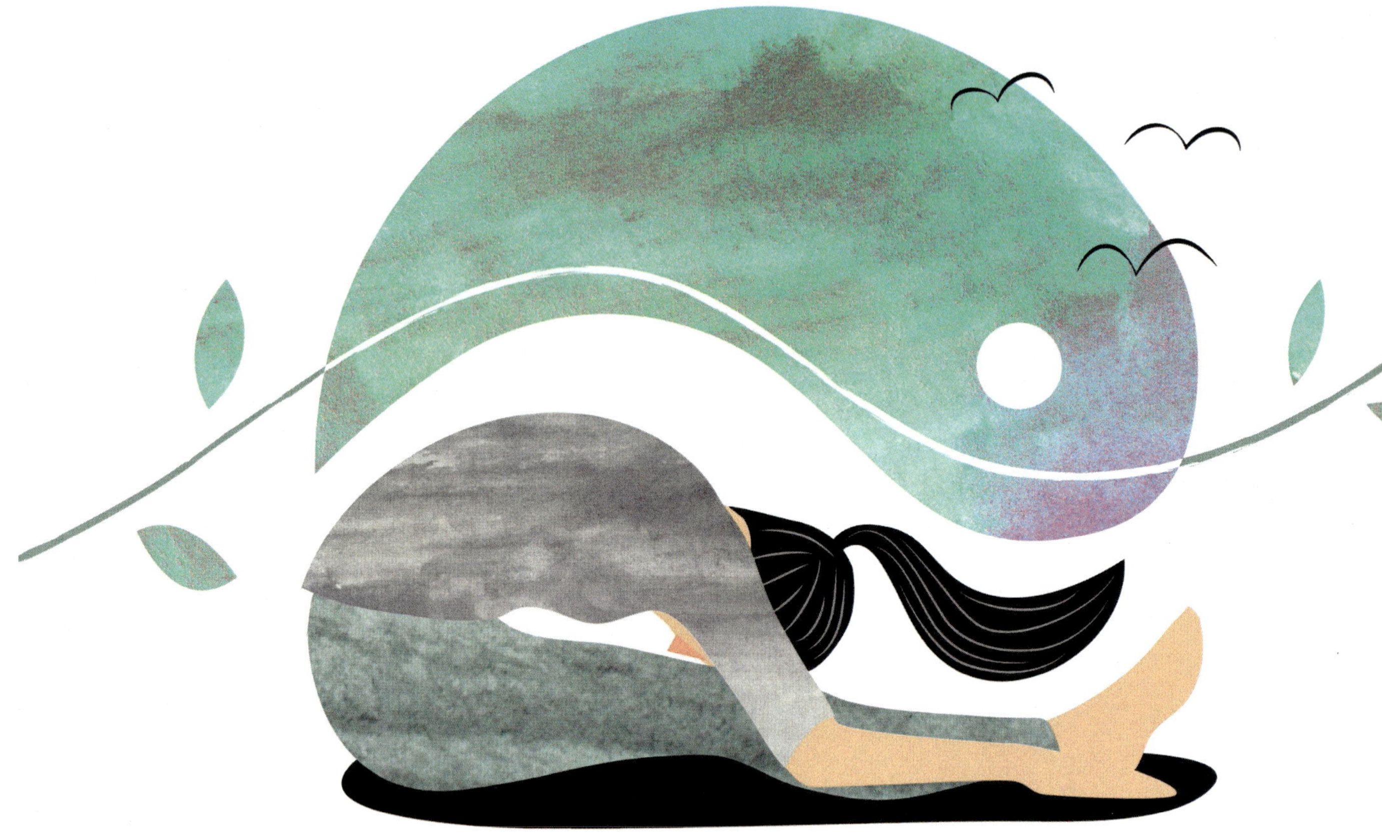

To have and to hold

Yin yoga encourages practitioners to spend more time exploring postures, which, in turn, can ease racing thoughts. Here, a yoga teacher explains how

What do we mean by yin?

With its roots in traditional Chinese medicine, yin-yang theory is a way of relating to the world. Yin is associated with the slower, cooler, calmer elements of life, while its opposite, yang, is more active and has warmer qualities. The key principle of the theory is one of achieving balance between these two ways of being, which in the case of humans means balance on a physical, mental, and emotional level.

Where yoga meets yin

The cool, calm, and steady qualities of yin are applied to yoga practice by slowing things down, remaining in postures for longer durations, and being mindful of any sensations and emotions that arise. Yin yoga suggests exploring poses for between three and five minutes. This is very different to many other forms of practice where postures are held for no longer than a minute, and especially fast-paced styles such as vinyasa and ashtanga, which flow from pose to pose without holding.

Yin yoga works with the body's connective tissues—deep layers of fascia, tendons, and ligaments that hold the body together and enable it to move. These can easily become tight and stiff with today's more sedentary jobs, but the stresses and strains of everyday life also take their toll.

According to traditional Chinese medicine, these same tissues are home to meridians—invisible lines of energy that run throughout the body, each corresponding with the organs and the various functions considered key to maintaining optimal health. Tapping into these meridians allows energy to flow freely, unblocking stagnation and helping to promote an improved sense of well-being.

By remaining in postures for extended durations, the tissues have time to relax and recognize the subtle signals being received. During this gentle exploration, they can also respond and adapt accordingly, through a process of release, rejuvenation, and hydration.

Yin yoga immersion

As well as a desire to share and teach my passion for yoga, I'm always keen to learn more from others. In my quest to understand more about the practice of yin yoga, I recently joined teacher and trainer Melissa Corazon for a weekend immersion in yin yoga. With a group of

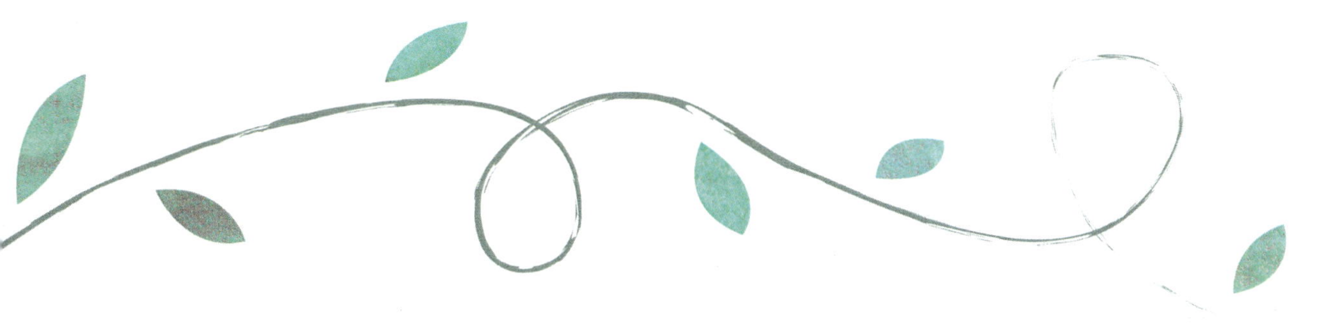

fellow yin-loving teachers, we experienced a thorough and enjoyable exploration of the practice in relative stillness, as we learned, lengthened, and laughed together. The physical, mental, and emotional effects of the immersion were amazing, lasting way beyond my reluctant departure on a sunny Sunday evening. Key to the course was gaining confidence with practicing and teaching in a much slower way, learning to become comfortable with quiet stillness, as opposed to filling time with words and movement. I'm a fan of mixing things up, and have since experienced great results by combining steady, fluid movements of mobilization and strengthening with deliciously long moments of quiet yin stillness.

Yin's "mindful edge"

As mentioned, the extended time spent in each position distinguishes yin from other forms of yoga, but there are other subtle variances. When moving into a position, yin calls for a "mindful edge"—a comfortable level of challenge that allows relaxation and a normal pattern of breath, which will differ depending on the flexibility of the practitioner. The use of props such as cushions, blankets, and yoga blocks is encouraged to support the body.

As yin yoga is particularly beneficial for less pliable muscles, it specifically targets the lower part of the body—the hips, pelvis, thighs, and lower back—all rich in these tougher connective tissues. The practice consists of a combination of 20 floor-based poses: lying down, seated, or kneeling. Although they closely resemble those from traditional hatha yoga, their names often differ and they are generally more descriptive of the look and feel of the pose and a somewhat different way of reaching it. Take the yin yoga caterpillar—while similar to the hatha paschimottanasana (known as seated forward fold in English), it differs in that it encourages a gentle rounding of the spine, as opposed to the straight, and therefore less-forgiving, spine of its hatha equivalent.

Sense of presence

The act of slowing things down creates a physical quality of stillness, which cultivates a sense of presence—physically and mentally—and helps to sharpen the brain, making it easier to focus and quieten the chatter in the mind. For some, yin yoga can also help to improve joint mobility and improve circulation—making it a great antidote to the stresses and strains of everyday life. Reflecting on the mind-body connection in yin yoga, Melissa says: "We gain a greater awareness and connection to our bodies. Through moving slowly and paying attention it can help us to be kind and compassionate to ourselves and our bodies. Accepting ourselves for how and who we are . . . which is immensely difficult, but through practice we can work toward it, slowly, slowly.'

Appeal of the calm

Yin yoga can also be the perfect complement to other activities and sports. It's an opportunity to relax and release after more dynamic or physically demanding pursuits such as running, cycling, or climbing. Melissa explains: "If you're used to doing a lot of movement, yin yoga is a completely different approach. Staying with the postures can be challenging but it's rewarding as you feel connected and centered and maybe even a bit more mobile afterward." Another perk of yin yoga is that there is no need for long or complicated routines. Even a short time in a single pose can help to change the course of a day.

Tini Wolfbeisser, a lawyer from Vienna, Austria, first experienced yin yoga while on vacation in Vietnam, where its calmness immediately appealed. "I was still fairly new to yoga but always appreciated calm poses that stretched my body, so I fell in love with this kind of yoga immediately," she says. Tini enjoys the energizing physical effects of her now regular yin yoga practice. "I love the prickling sensation and the energy inside my whole body afterward," she explains. "It feels like I've just had a really good massage and I can deeply relax and be fully content."

This slower form also gives time to tune into the breath, enabling it to become calmer and quieter as it settles to a deep, smooth, and steady rhythm. Calm breathing can also lead to a calm mind and Melissa sees this firsthand: "Students often report difficulty in relaxing and the practice of yin yoga has helped them with this. I often see a big change in them from when they come into the class compared to when they leave."

The simplicity and ease of yin yoga is part of its appeal and I couldn't agree more. For me, sometimes just a single pose practiced each morning—the swan (see overleaf)—helps me to start my day in a more mindful way. For Tini it provides calm closure from the daily demands of a challenging career: "Practicing yin yoga at home after a long day helps me to unwind from daily life and turn inward. It's amazing how it has such a positive effect." So, whether you choose to spend five minutes at home as a quiet caterpillar, or join a class with others, with regular practice you'll soon start to reap the physical, mental, and emotional rewards of this wonderful style.

SLEEPING SWAN

This pose provides a strong stretch for the hips and the front and back of the thighs, working with the meridians that help to promote a healthy flow of energy to the liver, kidneys, and gall bladder

- Start on the hands and knees in an all-fours position.
- Slide the right knee forward toward the right hand, slowly and carefully crossing the right foot and directing it toward the left hand—keeping the right foot flexed helps to protect the knee.
- Lengthen the left leg back, straightening it behind you with the top of the left foot facing down toward the mat.
- Take time to adjust the lower body so that the hips are even (you may need to position a blanket beneath the left thigh for this).
- Gently press the fingertips of both hands into the mat, extending the arms and lifting the heart.

This is swan pose.

- Find your mindful edge and remain here for one minute. Slowly transition to sleeping swan by walking the hands forward and lowering the upper body down to the mat, or onto a cushion or rolled-up blanket.

Hold for between two and three minutes.

WAKING THE SLEEPING SWAN

- Come out of the position by slowly walking the hands back to swan.
- Press down through the hands, to support the body, while drawing the left knee forward to return to the starting position.
- Repeat the above on the other side, starting by sliding the left knee forward.

As with all forms of movement, take great care to move within the limits of your body and stop immediately if any pain is experienced. Have some props to hand to make sure you can relax into the swan. There's no need for special yoga kit here—a trusty cushion or soft blanket are perfect.

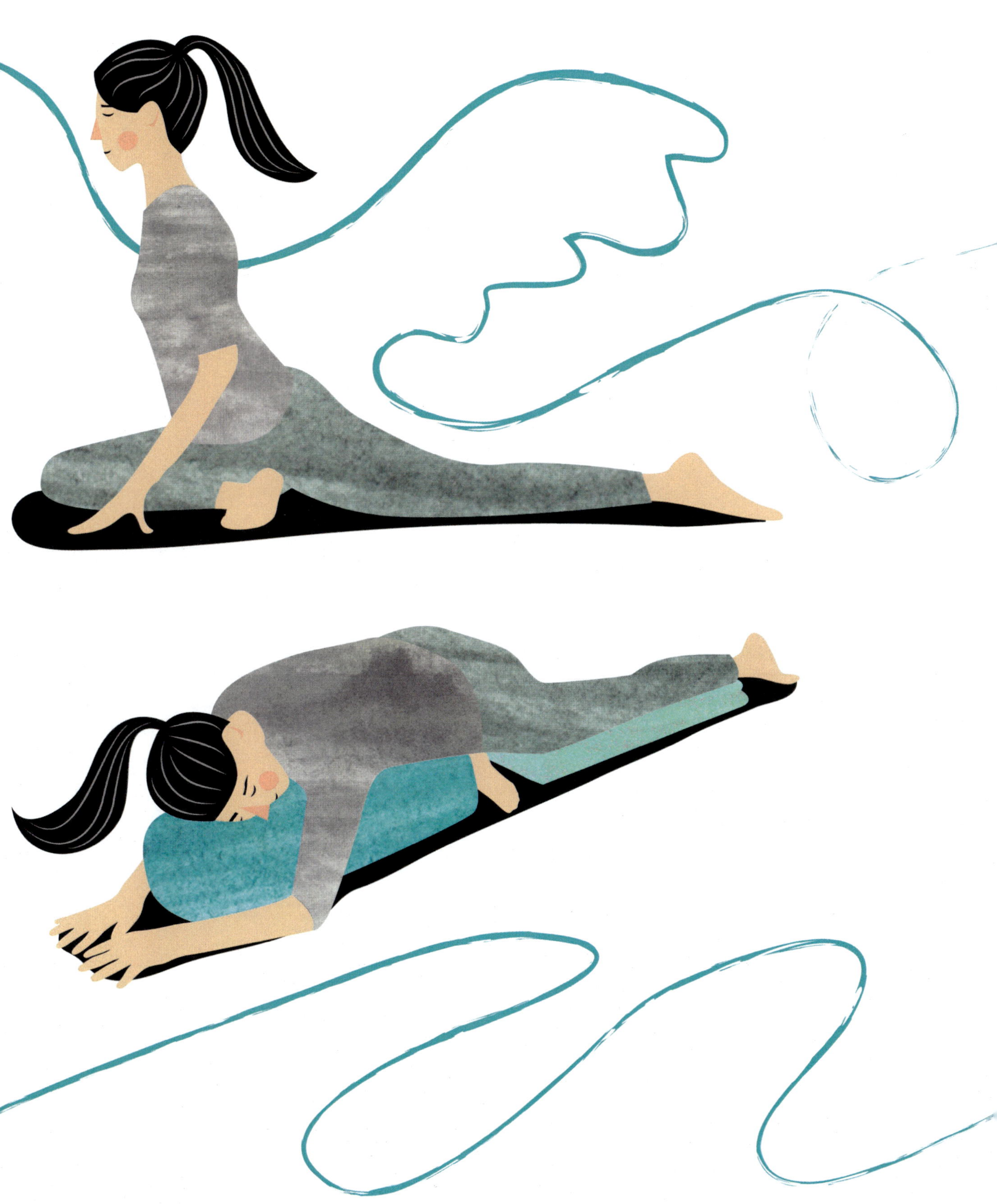

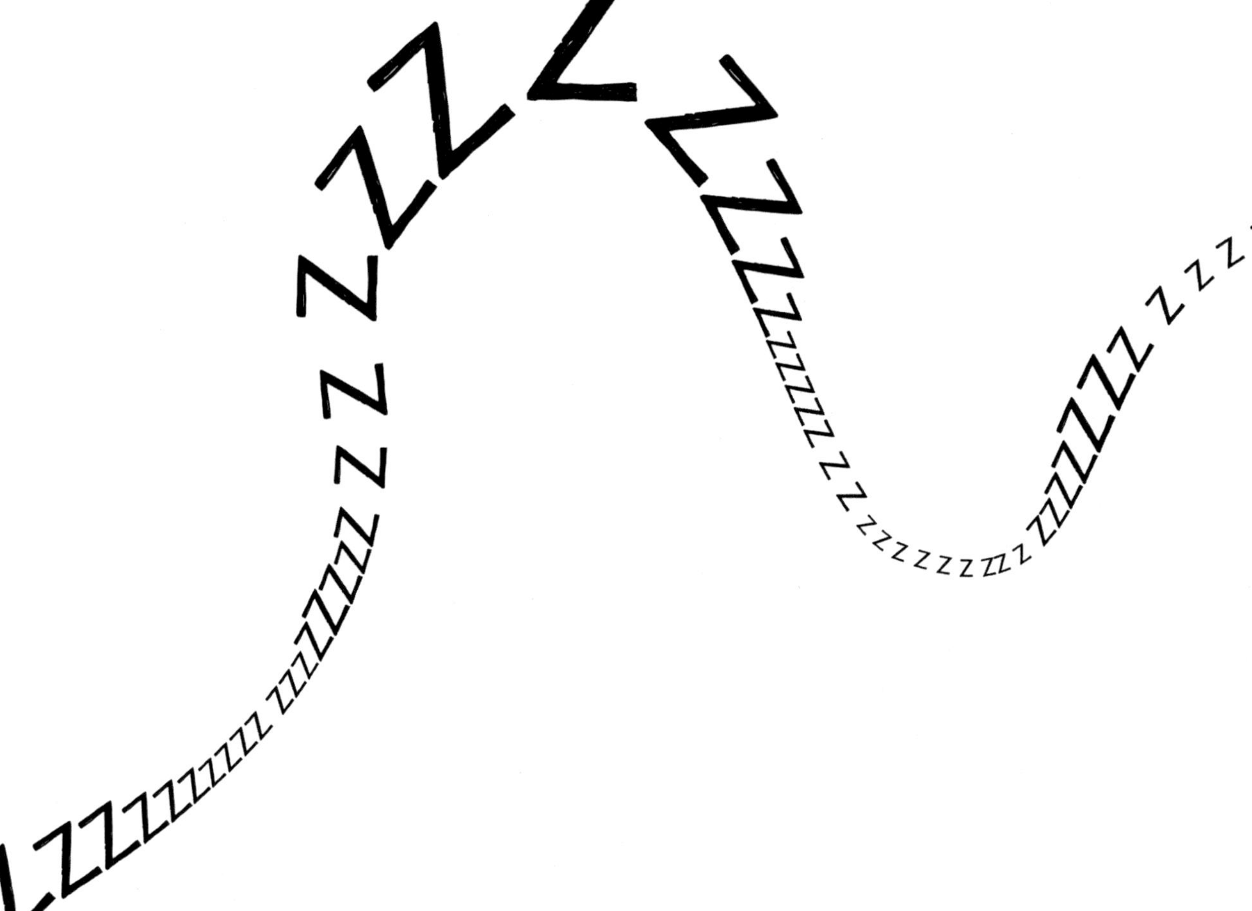

Pillow talk

What does your sleeping position say about your personality? From the fetus to the starfish, find out more about yours . . .

Your eyelids are getting heavy and, snuggled under your sheets, you relax into your mattress and pillows. You wriggle around the bed until you're comfortable. Within minutes (hopefully), you'll be asleep. But before you drift off, take a moment and notice your body's position.

"We usually find the best position for us by trial and error over the years," says Becki Houlston, a body-language expert and life coach who's also trained in neuro-linguistic programming (NLP). "Once we know what works for us, we rarely change it.

"But how we sleep is about much more than getting plenty of shut-eye," Becki explains. "We spend up to a third of our lives asleep, and how we position ourselves can tell us quite a lot about our personality and the way we operate."

Researchers have established six common sleeping positions, including the freefaller (sleeping on your front, as if you're parachuting from a height), and the soldier (lying flat on your back, with your arms by your side). So, how do you arrange yourself for sleep, and what does that say about the type of person you are during your waking hours? There are many interpretations. Here, based on her knowledge of body language, Becki gives us hers and offers a few helpful tips.

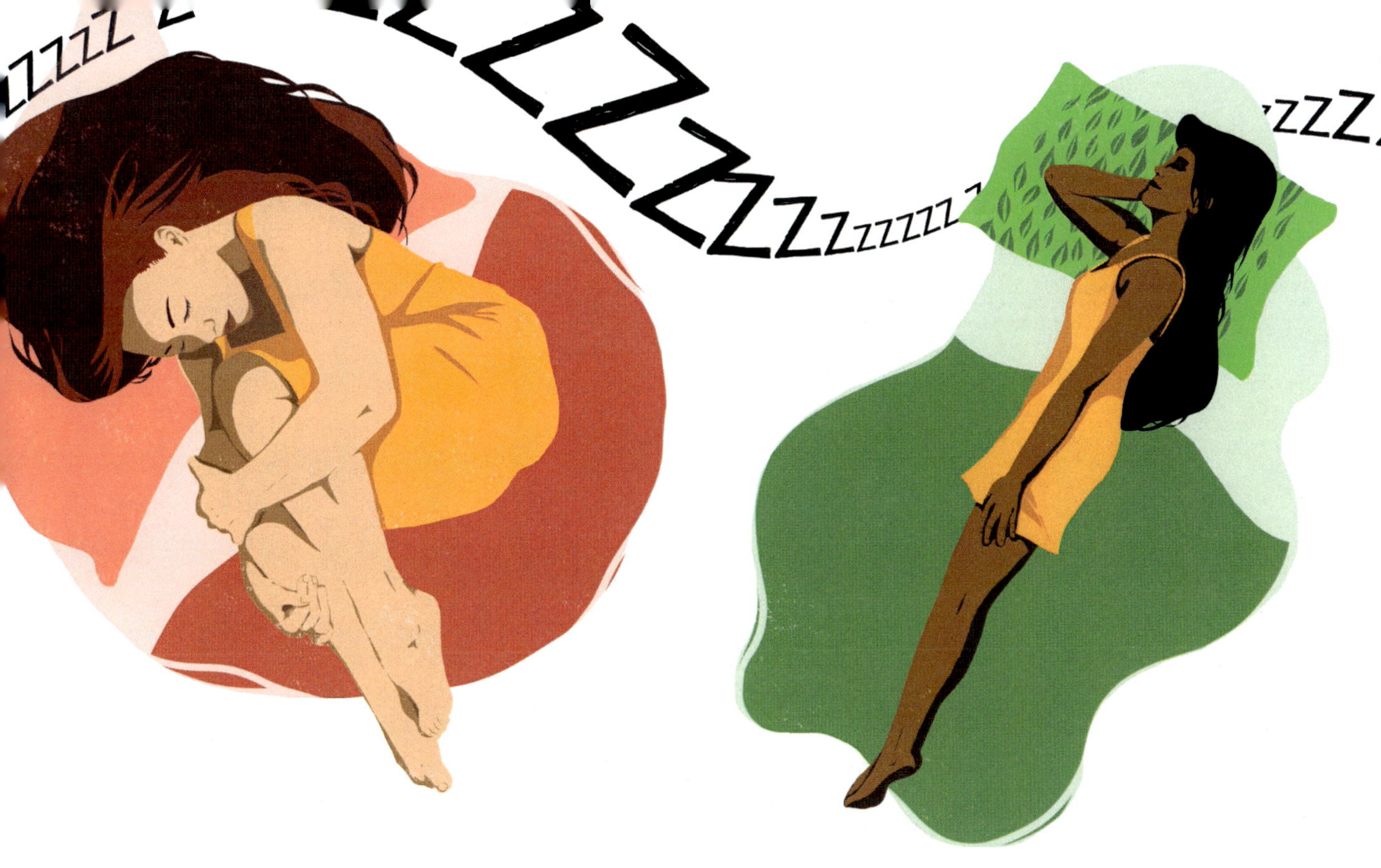

THE FETUS

You lie on your side, knees tucked up. You might swap sides in the night, but you tend to remain curled up, almost in a ball

Becki explains: "This is the earliest position we knew, so it's our nervous system's earliest memory. It's how we lay in our mother's womb, when we felt the world was safe. It's no surprise we associate this position with security."

Your personality

Security is important for the fetus sleeper. They try to meet their own needs, so they don't need to be dependent on others.

"The position itself is self-soothing, so people might get into it when they're worried or thinking a problem through. If they're ill, they won't involve others or ask for help with shopping or cooking. They try to do everything for themselves first, even if it's a struggle and others have offered assistance."

Tip: If you sleep in this position, consider taking up a new challenge, such as high-intensity interval training, a martial art, or mountaineering. "By engaging the physical, you will bring your mind and body together and re-engage the nervous system. This will give strength and in turn reduce the need for security."

THE LOG

You lie on one side, with your legs straight, and your top arm by your side

Becki explains: "Most doctors agree that sleeping on your left side is the best for your cardiovascular health. Pregnant women are advised to sleep on their left side because it's better for circulation and blood flow to the placenta. If you suffer from acid reflux, you're better sleeping on your left side too."

Your personality

"The log sleeper is grounded and they have a balance between their logical self and their feelings. They have a good sense of security and feel comfortable and secure. They know what they're doing and where they're going.

"If they get out of balance, they will overthink things, from the chat they had with a colleague at the vending machine, to a family party the coming weekend."

Tip: If you're overthinking things, write down everything on your mind or try doing a meditation before bed. "Relax about the nonessential things in life, even when they're threatening your sense of order. Ask yourself if the little things that are bothering you will matter in a few months' time."

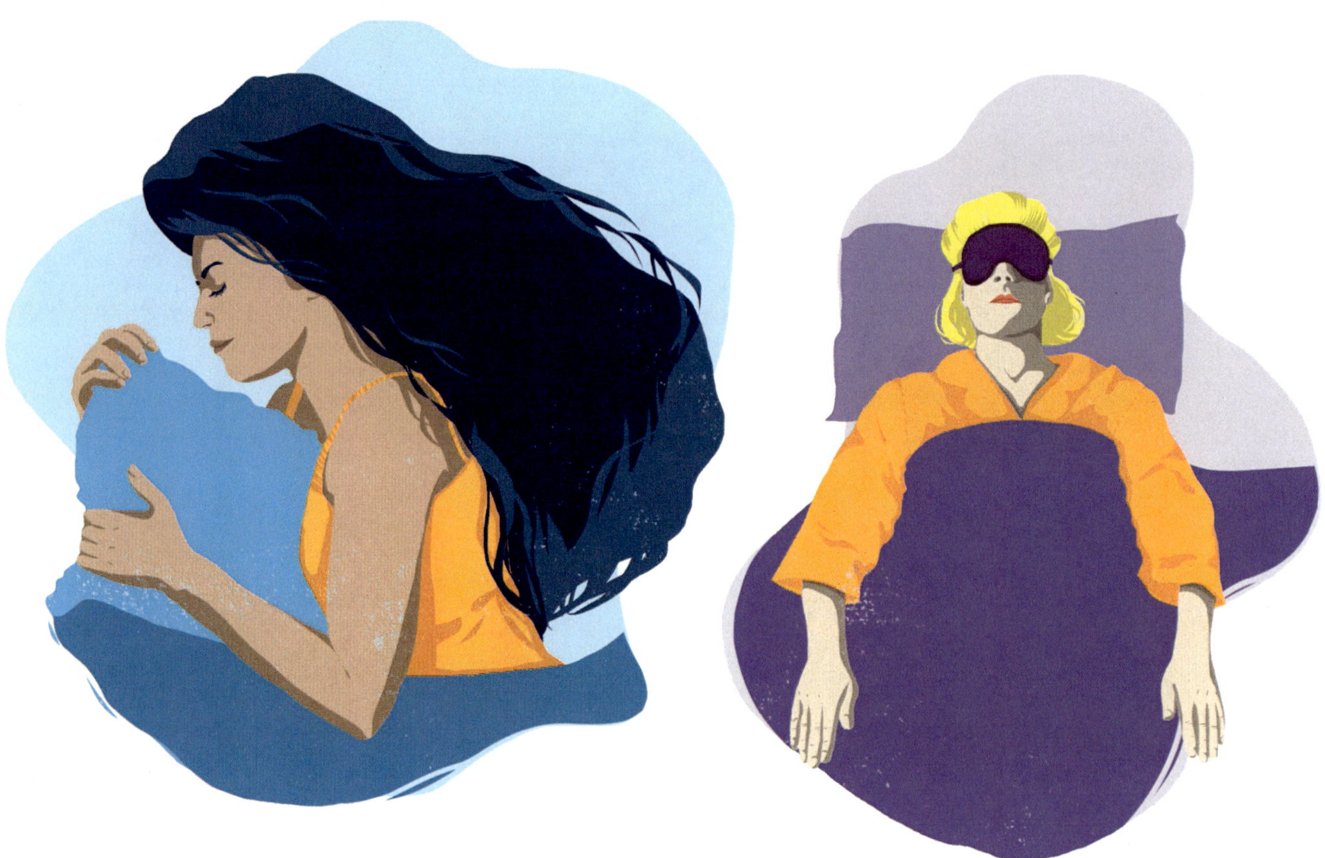

THE YEARNER

You sleep on one side, with your arms in front of you

Becki explains: "You lie as if you're cuddling a toy and, in reality, you might be holding a teddy bear or a pillow."

Your personality

"This person needs external validation, which means they need other people to praise them, thank them, and reassure them. Yearners need to be told they're good enough.

"Their inner child looks for security from the outside world and they can't get by without their friends.

"The yearner usually has a support network they can turn to for help. In fact, they sometimes ask for help as a knee-jerk reaction, before trying to resolve a problem for themselves."

Tip: Make sure it's not a one-way street when relying on friends and that you give back to them, too. "Ideally, build up your self-worth, so that your validation comes from inside and you don't have to go looking for it."

THE SOLDIER

You lie on your back, with your arms by your side

Becki explains: "This is the acceptance position in yoga, and we often use it for relaxation. Our weight is evenly distributed and it's good for the spine. Problems could arise if this sleeper is prone to snoring."

Your personality

The soldier is comfortable in their own skin.

"They're good as part of a team and can operate independently. They're also dependable and steady, and they like to achieve.

"They see sleep as functional and they won't read or watch television in bed. They just see their bed as a place to sleep."

Tip: Set time aside for self-care. "Sometimes, the soldier will be so busy getting things done, they'll forget to relax or have fun. They should also take time out to exercise as this will remove any negative energy they might have."

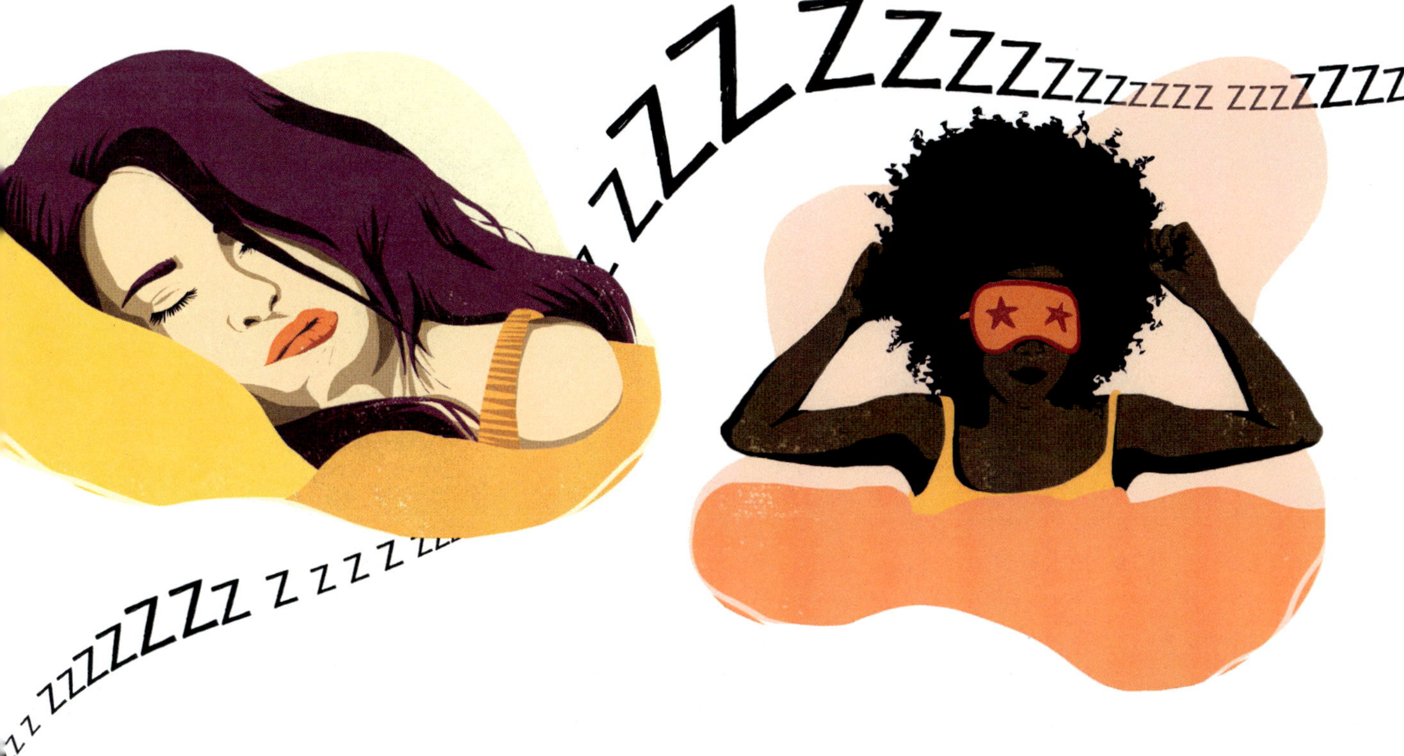

THE FREEFALLER

You sleep on your front, with your face in the pillow, or your head turned to one side

Becki explains: "This is a protective position. It's a throwback to primitive times because the person is protecting their organs yet looking out from the side to see if there are any threats coming their way."

Your personality

Freefallers have difficulty expressing themselves, especially what's important to them.

"They can shy away from conflict and prefer to gloss over disagreements to keep the peace.

"They often see the negative side of things and because of this, they're less trusting than they might be if they looked for positives. For example, if someone offers them help, the freefaller might question their motives. If they just saw it for what it was—an act of kindness—they might change their view of people.

"In relationships, they tend to hold back because they don't trust 100 percent. They often do what their partner wants to do, but every now and then they get resentful."

Tip: Start by working out what's important to you. "Once you understand what's important, you can start to tell others. It might be that you want 15 minutes at the end of the day to talk with your partner, uninterrupted by Facebook or the TV, or you might want help buying a car.If you start with little things, you can practice expressing yourself and then build up to bigger issues."

THE STARFISH

You sleep flat on your back with your arms above your head and your legs stretched out

Becki explains: "This position takes up a lot of space, and it's another one that's thought to be good for the spine."

Your personality

The starfish is open, trusting, and self-confident, but can be a little selfish.

"They can be funny and entertaining. They have sound internal validation and don't need others to tell them how good they are.

"The starfish is among life's organizers and they're enthusiastic. They come up with great ideas, like throwing a big family party to celebrate special birthdays, and often set the wheels in motion—choosing the day and drawing up a guest list. But they leave the hard work to other people.

"At work, if they're given a difficult task, they'll start the project and jot down a few ideas but soon hand it over to the team."

Tip: Recognize when you need to compromise. "Understand you're not always going to get things done your way and others won't want to dance to your tune all the time."

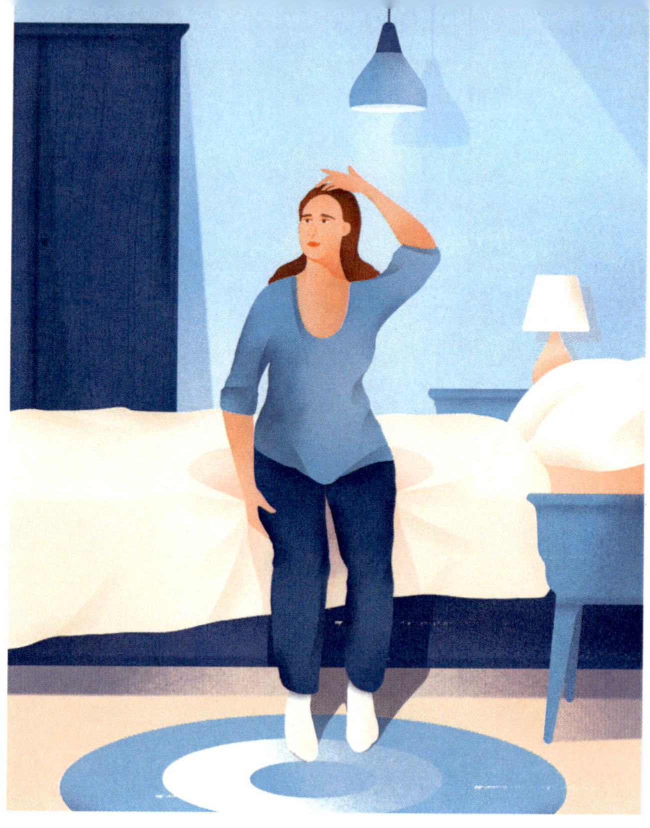

Release the tension

Whether you're suffering with sore, aching muscles or need to relax and destress, there are a number of simple self-massage techniques that can help

In recent times self-massage has come into its own and there are many techniques you can try to help ease and prevent minor aches, pains, and tension. Beata Aleksandrowicz is a massage expert who's written several books on the subject. She's trained spa masseurs worldwide and is a keen advocate of educating everyone on the power of touch, massage, and spiritual growth.

"Self-massage is easy to learn," she says. "It's a fantastic tool in an emergency, for sudden pain, for example. Or if you've stayed at the computer too long and feel aches in the wrist, neck, or shoulders. It can release tension and pain, and tide you over until you see a professional, if you need to. It can also be a valuable part of our daily ritual—offering five minutes of connection and the chance to be kind and generous to ourselves. We don't need to go to an ashram or a spa abroad. We can connect to and heal ourselves here and now."

Universal feelings

Beata became aware of the importance of touch after she spent time traveling in Africa, visiting Angola, Botswana, and Namibia, where she was acknowledged and initiated by healers. To explore the sensation of being deprived of touch, she worked with the Himba people of northern Namibia: "The Himba live on the open desert and they cover their bodies with okra paste to protect themselves from the elements," says Beata.

She performed massage and healing on them and found that "even though their skin is like armor because of the paste, their response when they were touched was very deep and profound." After this, she made *Touch of Trust*, a documentary that explores the ability to communicate through touch, which goes beyond cultural and language barriers.

"I've put my hands on thousands of people in the past 20 years. Massage is a tool of true transformation on a deeper level," she says. "It can, of course, address muscular or skeletal issues, but it also offers the chance to help you get back in touch with yourself."

Beata adds that self-massage might be a way of avoiding problems, too: "Done on a regular basis it can prevent the buildup of tension. It's an amazing way to celebrate yourself." But she stresses that self-massage and professional massage are different things. "You can't compare the receiving element. When you receive a massage, every system in the body is engaged. You can't massage every part of your body. Also, if you have a neck problem, self-massage might help, but you may need to see a specialist to address the underlying cause."

More than a treat

Massage is not just pampering, it can also be part of a health-boosting regime. The UK's NHS has recognized this in its advice to women who have had lymphedema following breast cancer, and offers guidelines on its website for lymph-boosting self-massage.

Beata agrees that opinions are beginning to change: "Massage can help balance hormone levels and blood flow, improve the lymphatic system, which is responsible for detoxification, and increase the release of endorphins, so people feel better."

Of course, not everyone feels comfortable with being touched by others and there are people around the world for whom self-massage could prove a useful alternative. Beata's experience is that "in hot countries, people tend to be more connected with their bodies . . . [whereas] in colder countries, where bodies are more covered, we're [in danger of] losing that connection if we don't make an effort."

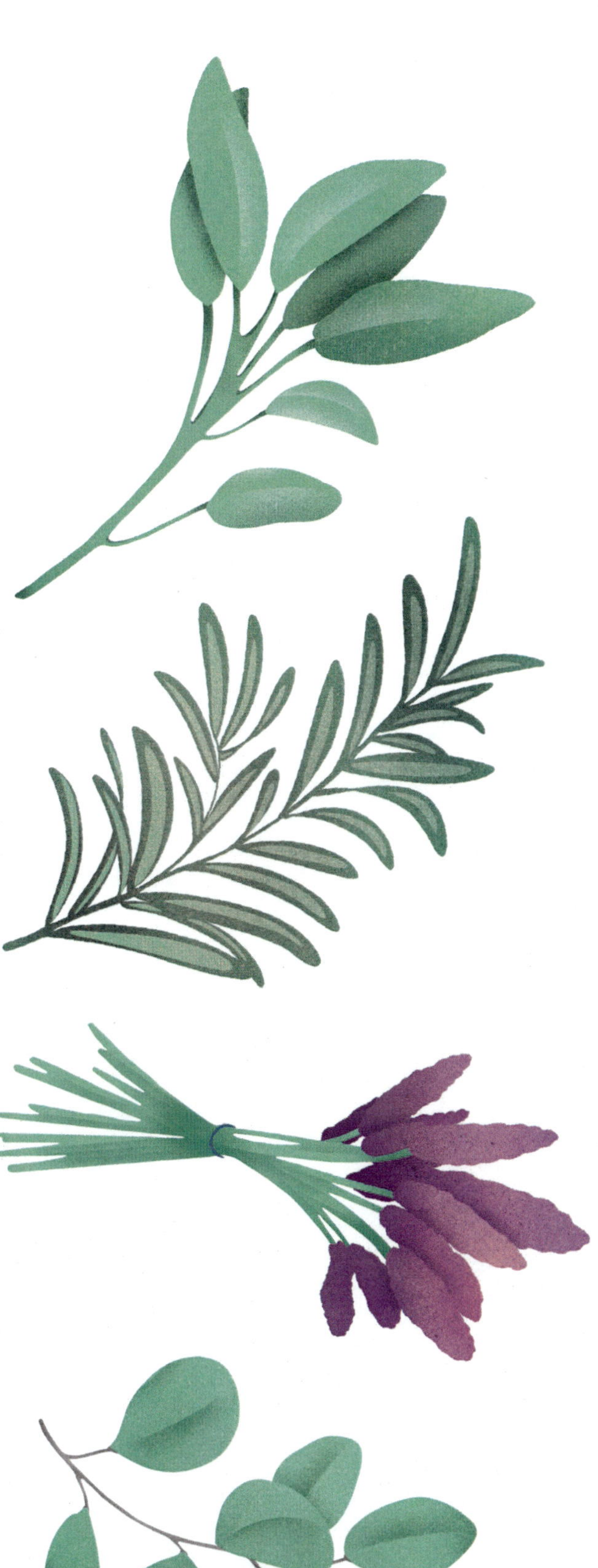

BEATA'S TIPS FOR SELF-MASSAGE

"The following sequences are great for combating the effects of a sedentary lifestyle, mild aches and pains, and general weariness. They are preventative techniques, designed to relieve temporary discomfort, tension, postural problems, or stiffness."

- Before starting, please read carefully the contraindications information, below. Women in the first three months of pregnancy are advised to avoid massage (and self-massage), owing to the risk of miscarriage. "We want to rule out any practice that could cause problems."

- "You can make your self-massage a ritual—light a candle, put on some nice music. Use any lotion or oil of your preference." This could be a light olive oil or almond oil with a few drops of your favorite essential oil added, or one that matches how you feel. For example, lavender is relaxing, eucalyptus is good for colds, rosemary and clary sage are warming.

- Make sure your room and the temperature are comfortable. A good time for a self-massage is after a bath because the muscles are more relaxed.

- Breathe deeply and steadily throughout the massages, which should also help to combat headaches and feelings of fatigue.

- As with all massages, work in a quiet, comfortable place, where you won't be disturbed or interrupted.

Once you're comfortable, try the self-massages over the page.

Contraindications

In certain circumstances you should avoid or be careful with self-massage:

- If you have painful bruises, fractures, or open wounds.
- If you suffer from serious and persistent back or neck pain.
- If you have a stomach upset.
- After a heavy meal (wait until at least an hour afterward before proceeding).
- If you have consumed alcohol or taken drugs.
- If you have a temperature (massage stimulates the body's metabolism, which can cause your temperature to rise even higher).
- If you have varicose veins. In this case, avoid pressure points and only massage the surrounding areas very lightly.
- It's advisable to avoid massage in the first three months of pregnancy. If you are, or think you might be, pregnant, do not practice self-massage (as per Beata's comments, above). From three months on, any massage of your lower back and abdomen should be very gentle. Seek professional advice before using essential oils. If you're in any doubt, see your primary care physician.

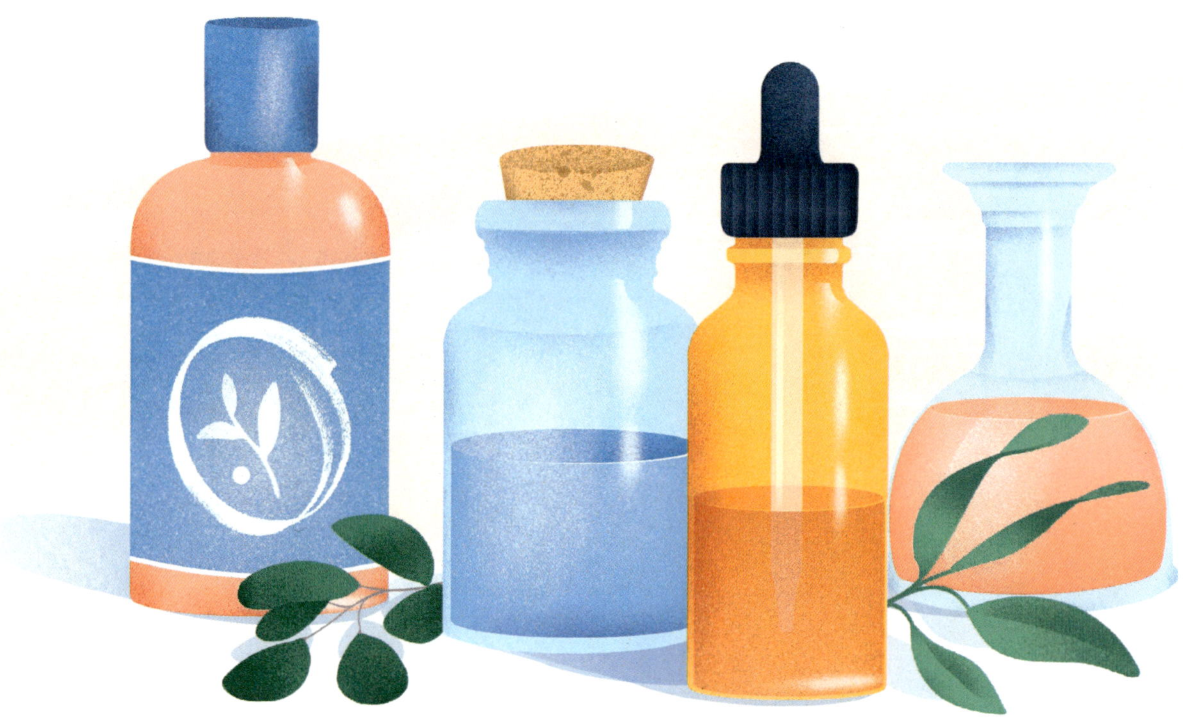

MORNING REFRESHER

Invigorating

Wake up physically and mentally when you haven't had enough sleep

- Sit on the side of the bed with your feet touching the floor. Relax your arms and make sure that you have a good connection between your feet and the surface underneath. Place your hands on your lap and close your eyes. Take a deep, slow breath. Gently, without any force, breathe out. Repeat three times.

- Put your right hand on your scalp, while the left one rests on your lap. Comb your fingers through the roots of your hair, close to the forehead, then close your fist, grasping as much hair as you can. Take a deep breath and, while breathing out, pull gently on the hair. Keep your fist very close to your scalp. Release.

- While taking another in-breath, reposition your right hand toward the back of your scalp, grasp as much hair as you can, and pull gently with the out-breath. Continue pulling and releasing your hair over the whole right side of your scalp. Pull firmly and rhythmically, so you can feel your scalp move. Use your left hand to work on the left side of your scalp.

- Place the fingers of both hands on your head and tap gently all over the scalp, breathing regularly. Imagine that heavy raindrops are falling on your head. Increase the speed of the tapping motion until you feel a pleasant warmth spreading all over your scalp. If you prefer, you can use relaxed fists, tapping gently, as an alternative to your fingers.

BODY ENERGIZER

Boosting

Use this technique to supply your whole body with fresh energy

- Stand with your arms relaxed and eyes closed, and breathe deeply several times. Open your eyes and, starting from the shoulder and moving down to the hand, cup your left arm rhythmically with the palm of your right hand. Move to a steady rhythm, matching your breathing to it. Repeat three times, change arms, and start again.

- Using your right palm, cup vigorously along your left shoulder as far back as you can reach, for 15 seconds. Do the same on the other shoulder, using your left palm. Make sure that you maintain the rhythm, and that your wrist stays loose. It's important that you use cupping only on the fleshy areas, avoiding bony parts.

- Move down, continuing the cupping on either side of your waist, then down along the hips, and up again toward the waist. Make sure that you stay on the sides of your body, avoiding the front, which is the site of your organs.

- Using both palms, cupping alternatively, work on your legs, one at a time, covering the top, both sides, and the back of the thighs. Work vigorously for at least 15 seconds, then move to the lower leg. Concentrate on the back half of the calf as the front is mostly bone. Cup in a steady rhythm for at least 15 seconds. Repeat on the other leg.

EVENING DE-STRESS

Soothing

A great way to finish the day and improve your sleep pattern

- You can either sit on a chair or on the edge of the bed. Relax and rest your right foot on your left knee. Slowly and gently, apply cream to the top and sole of your foot. Sandwich your foot between your hands, and make circles with both hands all over the foot, starting from your toes and sliding toward your ankle.

- Place both thumbs at the top of the sole, with fingers supporting the top of your foot. Press both thumbs into the sole and make three outward, deep, slow circles. Lift and move your thumbs to another point on your sole, press again, and make another three outward circles. Work all over the sole and heel, taking care to breathe regularly.

- Cup your heel in the palm of your left hand for support. Press your right thumb into your big toe. Make five slow circles in both directions, working on the whole surface of your big toe. Move to each of your other toes in turn and repeat the circles.

- Now, supporting your foot with your right hand, press your left thumb into the middle, top point of the sole. Slide down along this middle line to the edge of your heel, using your left thumb. Hold your foot between both hands, breathing deeply three times. Finally, repeat the whole massage sequence on your other foot.

SHOULDER STRETCH

Reinvigorating

Massage and stretch to release tension from your upper body

- Sit up straight and embrace yourself by placing each palm, with your fingers widely spread, as high up as possible on the outside of the opposite arm. Press your palms and fingers firmly into the upper arm muscles. Breathe out, squeezing and slowly massaging the muscles, using your fingers and middle edges of your palms.

- Slide your hands down your arms and embrace yourself just above the elbows. On the out-breath, squeeze the muscles and slowly massage them. Use your fingers for massaging the outer part of the muscles, and your thumbs for massaging the inner part. Repeat the first step—and this one—three times, massaging your arms in both positions on each occasion.

- Embrace yourself, reaching as far round the back as you can. On the out-breath, slowly stretch out your shoulder blades without lifting them. At the same time, bend your head slowly, creating a stretch along the spine and between the shoulder blades. Hold for a count of five. Slowly release.

- Place your arms behind your back, holding the right wrist with the left hand. Breathing out, slowly stretch your shoulders as far back as is comfortable, opening the chest and collarbones. Try to feel the shoulder blades touching each other. Hold for a count of five. Release.

For more information about Beata's treatments and teachings, visit beata.website.

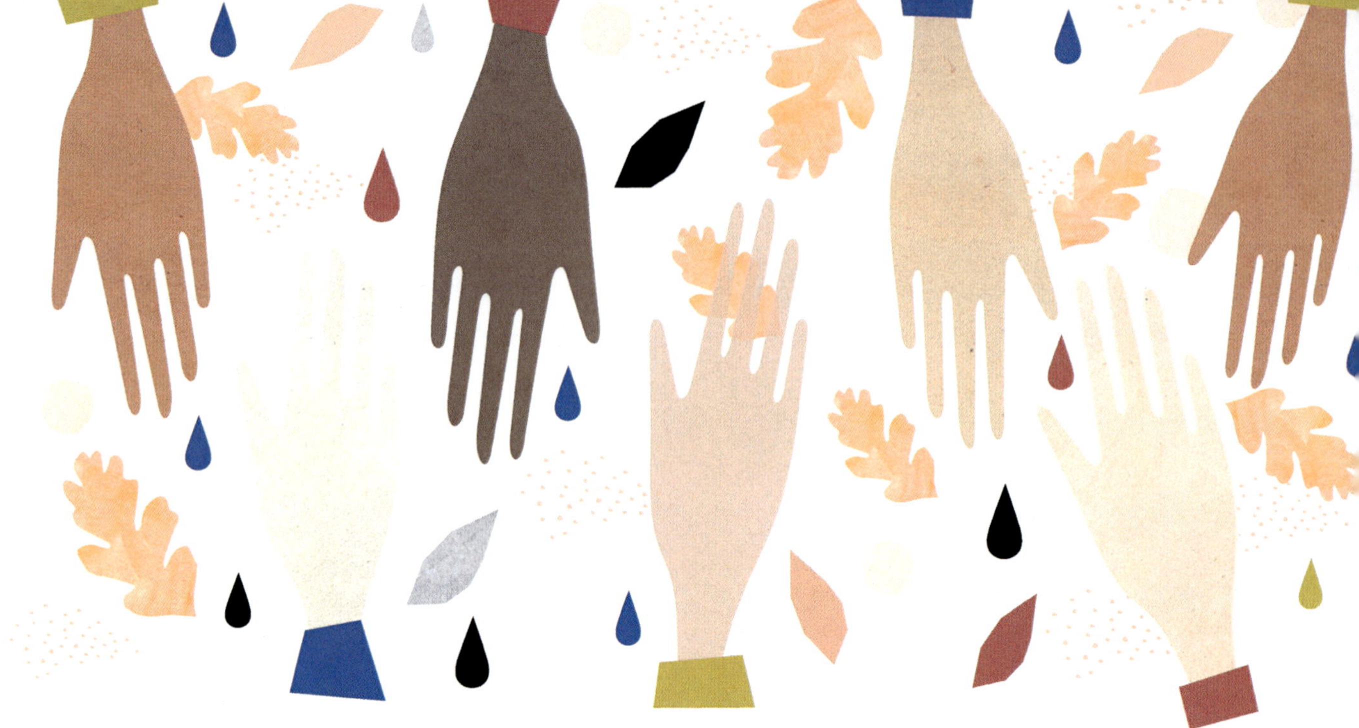

In good hands

It's time to give your hardest-working extremities the care they deserve

Hands are in almost constant use, engaged in untold daily tasks. From making the bed in the morning to preparing dinner in the evening, they're hard-working and largely uncomplaining. But apart from the occasional dab of hand lotion, how many of us give them the attention they need?

When you think about it, hands are remarkable for their strength and dexterity. It's been estimated that a quarter of the brain's motor cortex is devoted to hand-muscle function, enabling them to coordinate and perform complicated and meticulous tasks. Despite being such formidable tools, however, hands are more susceptible to the effects of environment, strain, knocks, cuts, and bruises than most other parts of the body.

Consider how many times a day they are immersed in water, exposed to heat, cold, or sunlight, or affected by chemicals or abrasives. How often do you carry heavy loads, perform repetitive tasks, or use your hands, fingers, and nails with force to tackle tricky jobs?

Handle with care

Despite appearing robust, the skin on the top of hands tends to be thin and has few moisture-regulating sebaceous glands, which means the skin here can become dry, irritated, chapped, and leathery. Over time, the muscles, ligaments, and joints in the hands reveal the impact of everyday use, and they are one of the first parts of the body to show signs of aging. To keep hands healthy and in reasonable shape, it's worth taking time to include them in your daily self-care routine. This isn't about gels, varnishes, or tips, it's about protecting your hands—sparing them from unnecessary environmental damage, overuse, and neglect—so that they stay nimble and in good shape for longer. It's partly about moisturizer and a nail file, but it's also about not putting your hands under more stress than is necessary.

Benefits of exercise

Lynn Houghton, a clinical specialist in hand therapy, explains that, with aging, tendons might not glide as smoothly and wear and tear can cause joint deterioration: "The joint at the base of our thumb allows flexibility to pinch and grasp. Normal use of the hand puts large forces through this joint, particularly pinching activities, and some 22 percent of people aged 50 and above develop basal thumb osteoarthritis. These deteriorative changes can cause pain, swelling, and a reduced range of movement. Everyday activities, such as writing, unscrewing jars and opening cans, might aggravate symptoms."

Taking extra care of your hands and exercising them will help to maintain muscle tone and hand mobility. "Exercise has many benefits. It can help ease stiffness, improve movement, and strengthen muscles," Lynn explains. "Tendon glides, or other specific hand exercises, may be prescribed by a hand therapist, while customized splints can provide support. Aids such as spring-loaded scissors, electric jar openers, key turners, and pen grips distribute pressure and reduce stress on joints. Also, switching tasks and pacing yourself helps to avoid hand fatigue."

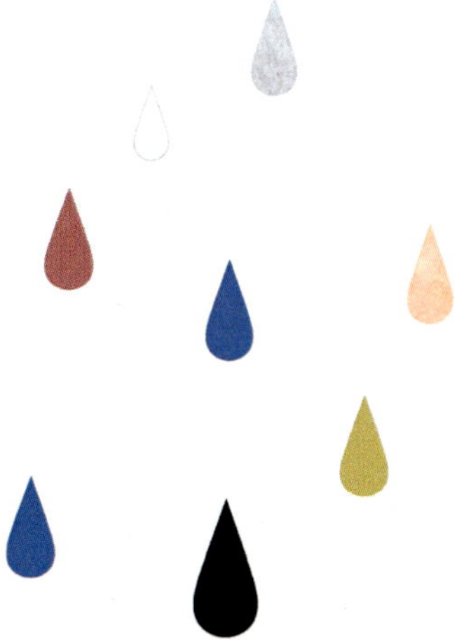

HOW TO CARE FOR YOUR HANDS

Use natural soap

Appropriate handwashing (before and after contact with food, after using the toilet, visiting clinical settings) is a good defense against bacteria and viruses, but washing frequently can strip skin of vital natural oils and cause dryness or irritation. Choose a natural, gentle hand soap—these will remove viruses just as well as antibacterial soaps.

Wear gloves

A cozy pair of gloves will keep your hands warm on winter days. It's also a good idea to wear suitable environmentally-friendly gloves for domestic, gardening, or work-based duties, especially if you're frequently immersing your hands in water, using harsh detergents, or doing work that's tough on your skin. Choose washing-up and gardening gloves that are kinder to you and the planet. Look out for household gloves that are compostable and made from FSC-certified natural rubber sourced from a responsibly managed plantation.

Moisturize and massage

Choose a good-quality, organic hand cream that hydrates, softens, and protects, and use it at least twice a day.

Exercise

Take a few moments to gently exercise your hands, which will improve circulation and mobility. For example:

- Make a light fist with each hand and release, expanding the fingers.
- On each hand, bend each finger in turn toward the palm. Hold for a few seconds and release.
- Lay palms flat on a table, and raise each finger one at a time.
  Repeat each exercise several times.

Rest

If you do repetitive tasks that exert pressure on hands and wrists, remember to take regular short breaks throughout the day. This helps to avoid repetitive-strain injuries.

Special treatment

You may have heard of reflexology for the feet, but did you know you can also benefit from reflexology on your hands? This ancient healing practice targets specific areas of the body, by applying pressure to certain points, and is relaxing and therapeutic. If you have any concerns about your hands, however, consult a qualified specialist first.

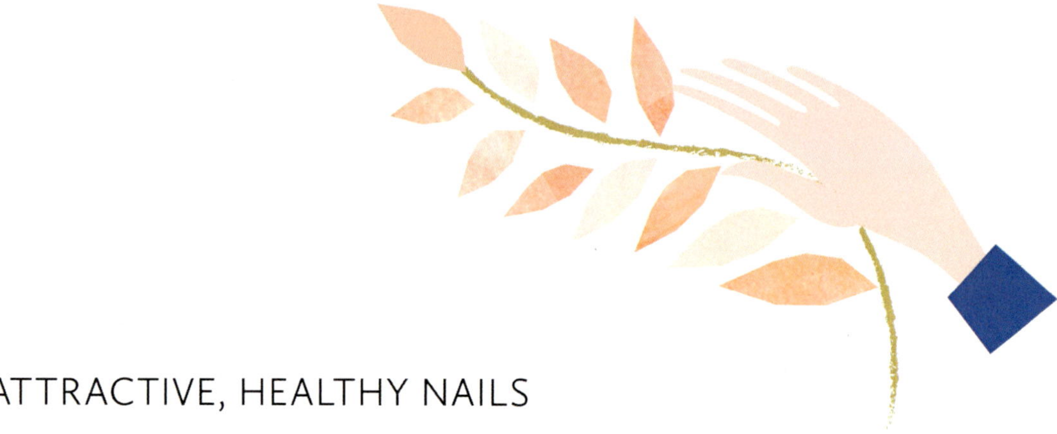

ATTRACTIVE, HEALTHY NAILS

- Nails can harbor germs, so keep them clean. Use a nail brush to remove dirt then dip your fingertips into a bowl of warm water, containing two tablespoons of apple cider vinegar or two drops of lemon oil, for a deeper clean.
- Trim your nails after a bath or hand soak as they'll be easier to cut. Use an emery board to shape and slightly round the nails at the corners.
- Although wearing artificial nails, varnish, or nail art can bring a touch of elegance and style to your hands, going natural whenever possible lets nails breathe and avoids discoloration or damage. But there's another good reason—nail condition is an effective indicator of general health. For example, nails that are brittle or show white spots, ridges, or discoloration might suggest a dietary imbalance, allergy, or possible health issues. Keeping nails natural means you can see and check anything unusual.
- Do you wear false nails to hide bitten ones? If you're a nail-biter, try to focus on breaking the habit. On average, fingernails can grow up to four inches per year, so visualize your nails growing strong, healthy, and beautiful.
- Once a month, give your nails and cuticles a conditioning soak (see recipe, right). And when you moisturize your hands, remember to massage the lotion into the nails, too.
- Many people take care of their own nails, trimming and filing them when needed, but consider treating yourself to a professional manicure once in a while, to give your nails special attention.

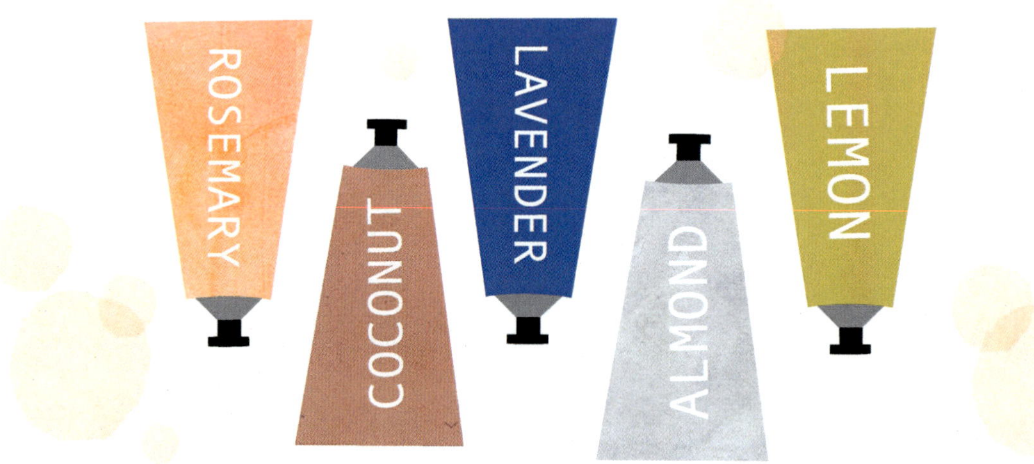

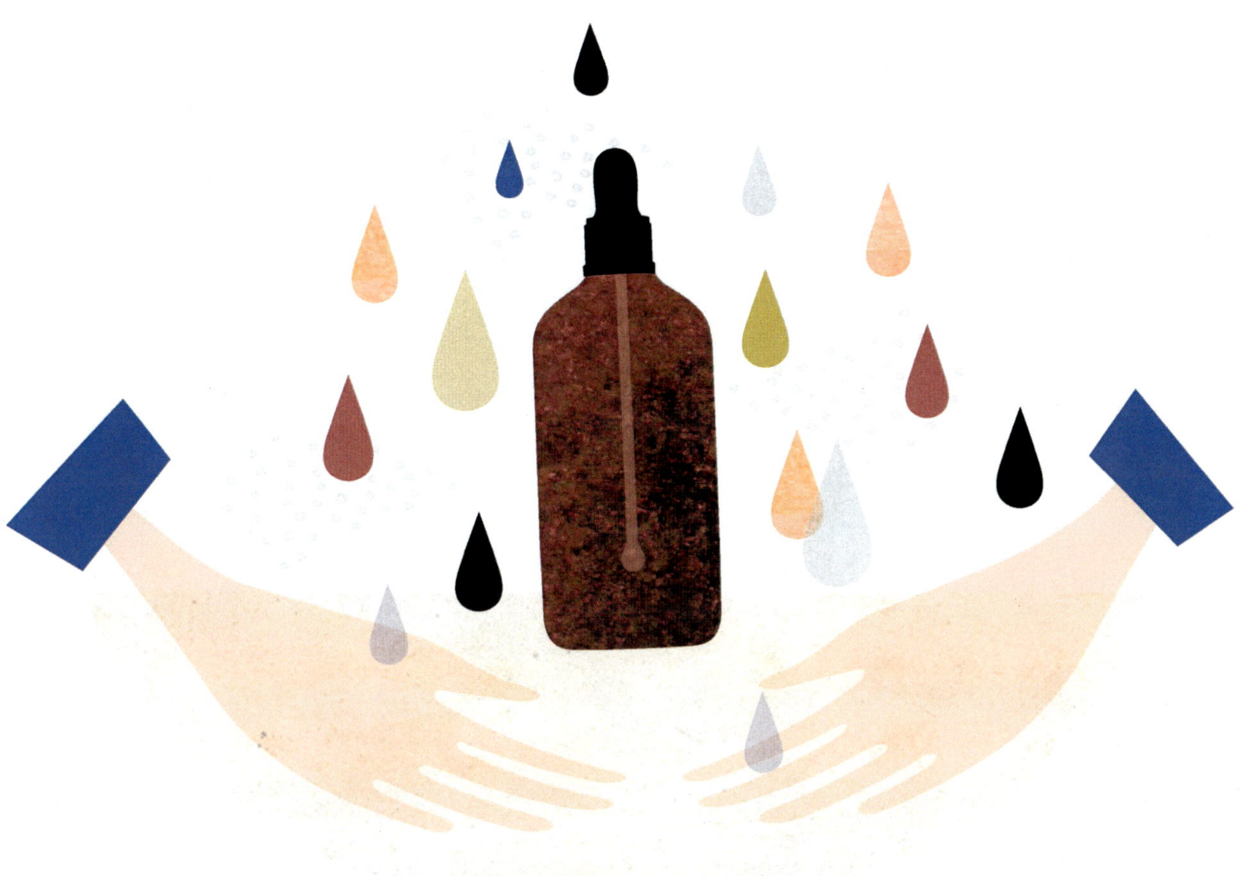

NATURAL TREATS

Hand-care scrub

Ingredients:

- 1 tbsp coconut oil
- 3 drops frankincense oil
- 2 drops lemon juice
- 1 tsp sea salt

Combine the ingredients in a small bowl and rub the scrub over the backs and palms of the hands. Pay attention to wrists, fingers, and thumbs. Rinse and dry gently and thoroughly before moisturizing. Exfoliating every few weeks with a natural hand-care scrub will help to remove dead skin and improve circulation. This scrub is gentle, but effective, and your hands will feel softer afterward.

Nail-conditioning soak

Ingredients:

- 4 tbsp olive oil
- 5 drops lemon oil
- 3 drops lavender oil
- 2 drops rosemary oil

Combine the ingredients. Buff and then soak the fingernails in the mixture for about 10 minutes. Rinse and pat dry before moisturizing. This will help to maintain clean, healthy nails and ease torn or dry cuticles. It can also help to ward off fungal or bacterial infection.

Hand mask

Ingredients:

- 3 tbsp fine rolled oats
- 2 tbsp rose water
- 2 tbsp baking soda
- 2 tsp almond oil

Mix all the ingredients and heat gently until just warm (be careful not to let the mixture overheat or boil). Apply the warm mask to your hands and then wrap them up in a clean towel. Leave until the mask is cool and gently rinse away the mixture. Pat dry and apply hand lotion.

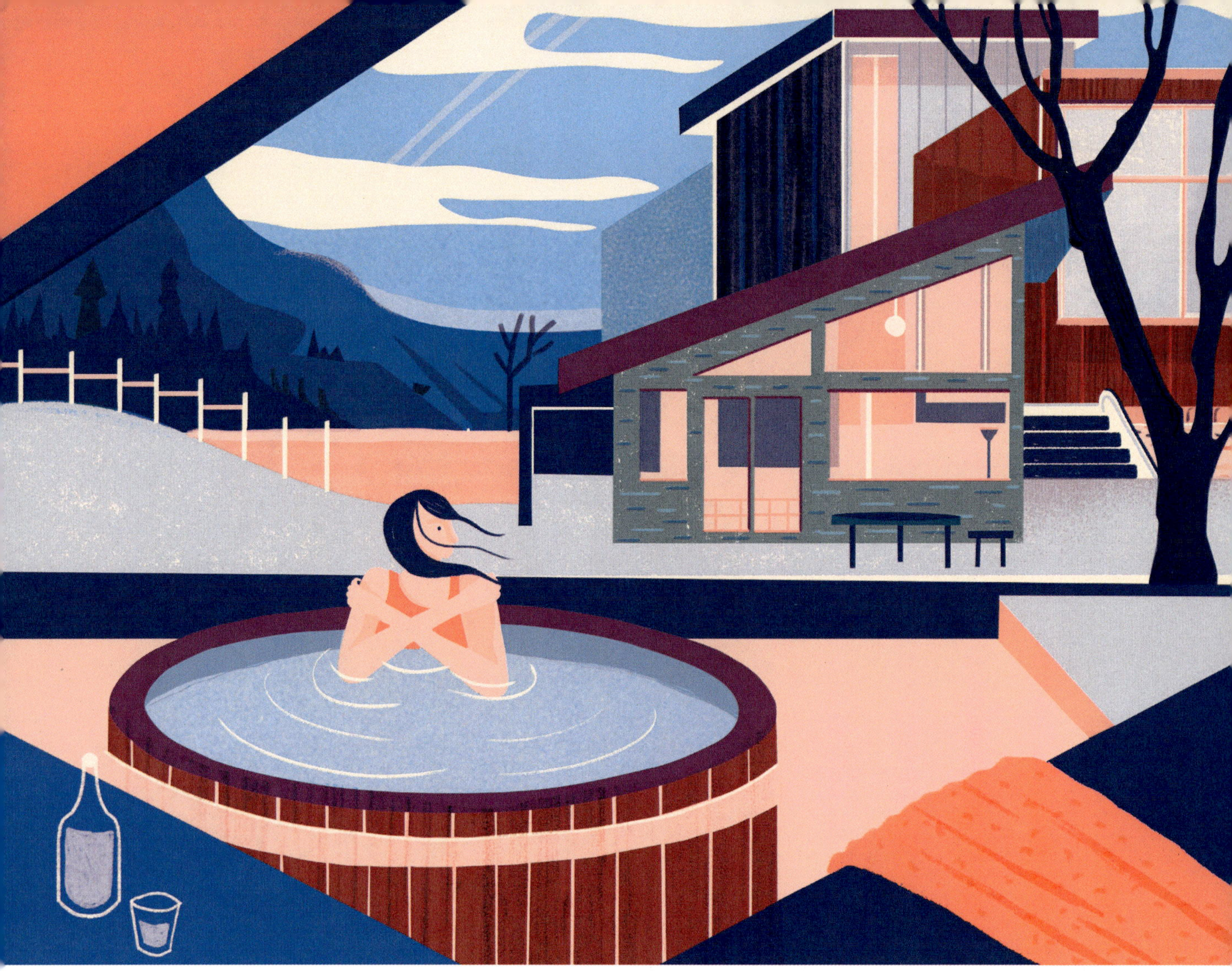

The big chill

Could taking a plunge in cold water or having an ice-cold shower first thing every morning boost health and self-esteem?

Living in rural Ireland brings with it a certain love affair with nature. It would be virtually impossible to inhabit this part of the world without developing a strong relationship with the surroundings. The sea, the fields, the bracken all come together to create a sometimes barren but enchanting landscape that reaches into the heart and captivates the soul.

I'd like to think of myself as having a strong constitution and winter is an opportunity to connect to that wild side. This year, I wanted to keep that spirit alive for the long winter months, to tap into something that would both challenge and invigorate, something that would reinforce my connection with wildness.

From a young age, the Atlantic has always felt like home and when I swim and my body hits the water I feel a return to self and a sense of relief. I wanted to maintain that feeling of invigoration, of the body being kickstarted into action—cogs running and whistles blowing—beyond the summer. There's also the clarity of mind that comes after a swim and that delicious feeling of your body warming up from the inside.

This prompted my decision to embark on a 30-day cold-water experience to see if my body would welcome or shun this pretty brutal practice. What I wasn't prepared for was the positive effect on my mental health. I'd felt this idea brewing in me for a while and couldn't ignore it any longer. You could describe it as my body knowing exactly what it needed or it could have been remnants from articles and books I'd read on the effectiveness of cold-water therapy. Wherever the inspiration came from, I found myself on

"I'd done my research and I knew that if I kept my awareness on my breathing and didn't panic, this could feel effortless"

a miserable drizzly morning, walking out to my hot tub (filled with ice-cold water) for a dip. My feet were already numb and in pain from the walk and my resolve was slowly fading with each step.

Breathing deeply was what I was relying on to keep me from running away. As I took my robe off and felt the cold wind on my skin, my mind was screaming run, don't do this, it's going to hurt and be so cold. But I had already researched the subject and felt reassured that if I kept my awareness on my breathing and didn't panic, this could feel effortless. So, in I went. It was cold. It did hurt. But my breathing kept me from running off and, after a minute, I felt my body relax. I stepped out and walked back into my warm home and carried on with my day.

From that day on, I committed to either a cold shower or a cold plunge in the tub. I noticed how quickly my mind tried to convince me not to do it. First thing in the morning, when you're drowsy and warm from sleep, the last thing your body wants to do is be immersed in cold water. I always took note of how I felt after. Accomplished. Proud. Energized. Clear.

I was facing my fear and going through with it, choosing not to let my mind dictate my actions and focusing on my breathing—this allowed me to connect to the present moment and prevented my fear from taking control.

This experience, especially practiced daily and first thing, provides a boost that can be carried throughout the day. And it's about so much more than what it does for you physically—it's as though facing something uncomfortable and difficult each morning paved the way to tackle other fearful tasks.

After 30 days there was no way I could stop. By April, I reached day 60. Sometimes it feels easier to face than others, but mostly it's dependent on my mind and if I give in to the ego and take overthinking seriously. For the most part, I love it.

If you are, or think you might be pregnant, or if you have any existing medical conditions or any health concerns, please talk to your primary care physician or medical advisor before taking cold showers or going cold-water swimming. Always have warm, dry clothes nearby after taking a cold dip.

NEED MORE CONVINCING?

Here are five things I learned from 30 days of cold showers

1. You can be scared of something and do it anyway.
2. Your mind is a powerful tool for distraction. Don't let it convince you that you cannot physically do something.
3. A cold shower gets you present. Deep breathing makes you regain control and stay in the moment even if that moment is somewhat painful. It's a powerful lesson.
4. Your body gets used to it and actually starts to crave the cold. Yes, that might seem impossible but I cannot wait for cold showers now. They are invigorating.
5. You become proud of yourself and this improves self-confidence. Even something as simple as a cold shower sends the message that you can do anything. I made some big decisions during my first month of cold showers and that was boosted by facing my fear every morning and smashing through it.

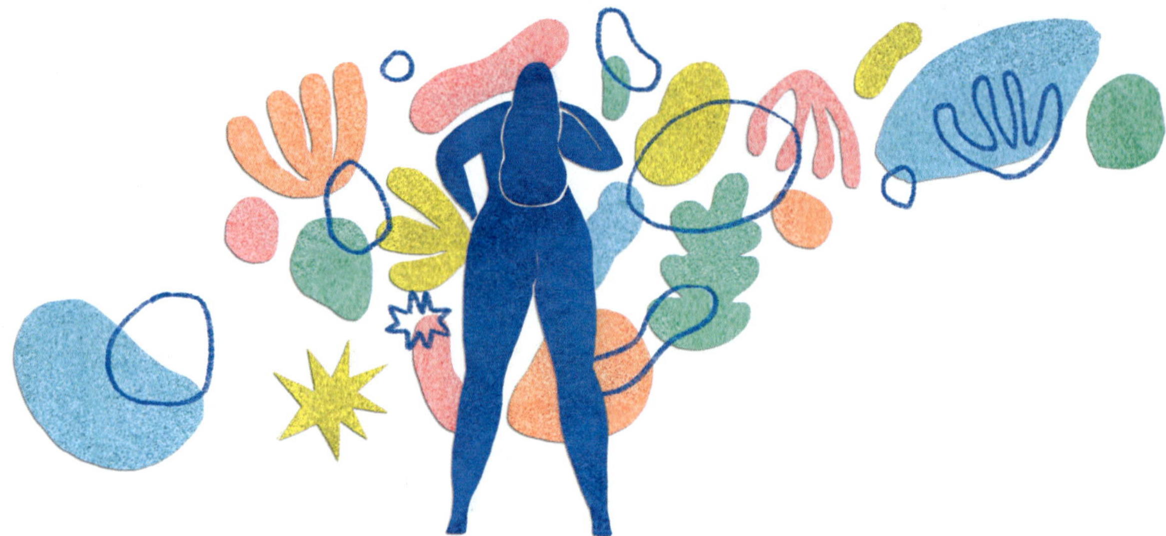

Spoilt for choice

It's often regarded as advantageous, but having too many options can cloud your judgment, making it difficult to reach decisions. Thankfully, there's a way round it

Many people have experienced it. Those moments of paralysis and fear when faced with difficult life decisions. Weighing up the pros and cons of what can seem an overwhelming number of choices and possible consequences can frequently lead to dread, anxiety, or even inertia.

But what if there was a better way to look at the situation? Scientists have established that by letting go of the belief that there's one right decision, and investing in the process of making choices, you can learn more about yourself and explore new and unimagined possibilities.

Fast and slow thinking

The study of decision-making is a relatively recent one, with Nobel Prize-winning psychologist Daniel Kahneman being a pioneer in the field. In his book, *Thinking, Fast and Slow*, he explores two different ways the brain forms thoughts, how each affects decision-making, and why both can lead to error.

Fast thinking is the most dominant mode of decision-making. Automatic, sensory, and predictive, these decisions are frequently based on past experiences, heuristics (simple mental processes, when an individual focuses on the most relevant aspects of a situation to find a solution), and gut instinct. Gaps in information are overlooked, quick conclusions are made, with something that maintains the status quo often emerging as the preferred option. The busier and more time-constrained people are, the more likely they are to default to this type of thinking.

By comparison, slow thinking is more deliberate, reflective, and effortful. Triggered in response to new situations and events, different options are investigated, new information and knowledge is sought, and even opposite views adopted, to test certain assumptions. This is not to say that slow is better than fast. Intuitive thinking is powerful, rich, and complex. "[It's] the origin of much that we do wrong, but also of most that we do right," says Kahneman. However, when it comes to making difficult decisions, slow thinking has the potential to help identify and explore new possibilities and choices. It can curb default biases to bring new insight. The challenge is to slow down enough to let this kind of thinking emerge.

Multiple choices

Decisions about where to live, parenting, career, retirement, and whether to end an important relationship are some of the life challenges people face. Then there's the more routine type of decision-making that we carry out every day. Recent studies by psychologists indicate that people want less choice, not more.

In their article, *When Choice Is Demotivating: Can One Desire too Much of a Good Thing?*, professors Sheena Iyengar and Mark Lepper of Columbia and Stanford University respectively, share their study of supermarket shopping and the impact of choice on decision-making.

Over two Saturdays, shoppers were offered a range of jams to sample, with the incentive of a $1 discount for each jar purchased. In experiment one, six varieties were displayed; in the second, 24. Unsurprisingly, more people were attracted to the 24-variety stall and tasted the jams on offer. However, when it came to purchasing, customers were almost 10 times more likely to buy from the first experiment than from the second, with the larger selection.

While this test may seem trivial when compared with difficult life decisions, the results offer useful insights into choice preferences. Of the findings, the professors write that they "challenge a fundamental assumption underlying classic theories of human motivation and rational choice

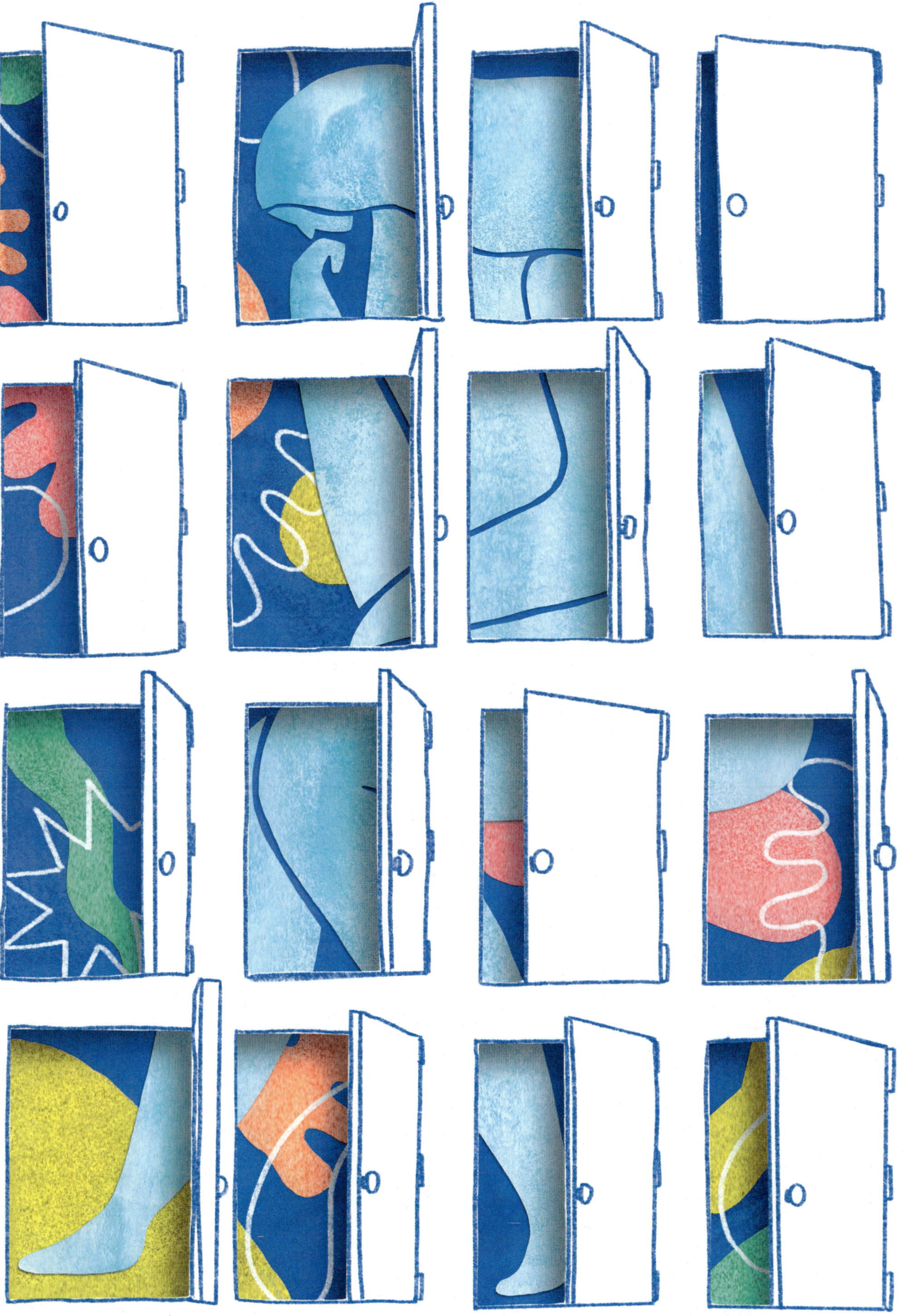

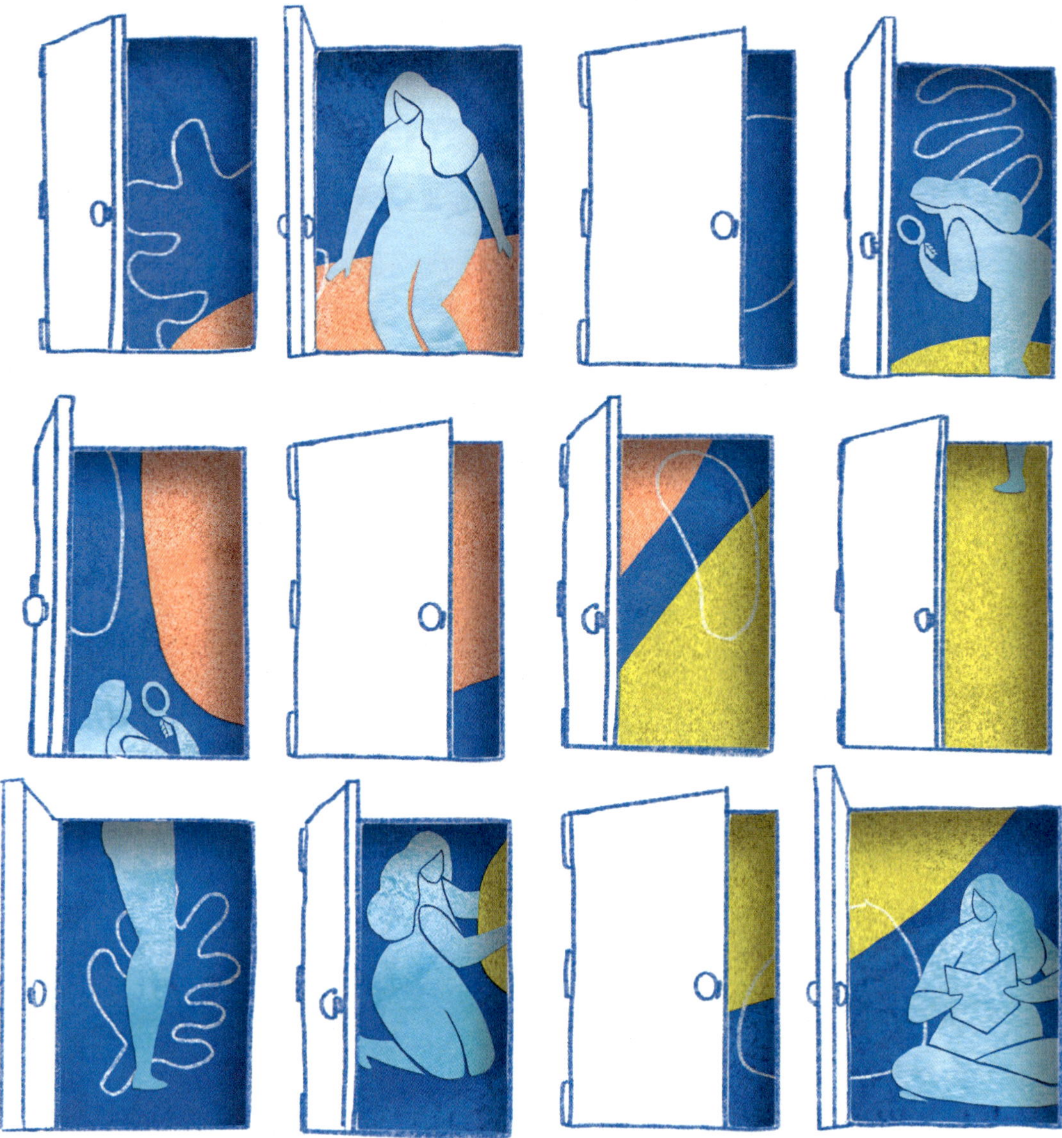

that having more, rather than fewer, choices is necessarily more desirable and intrinsically motivating."

Multiply this scenario by 70—the average number of decisions Sheena believes people make daily—and it's easier to understand what psychologists call "choice overload." In his book, *The Paradox of Choice*, psychologist Barry Schwartz argues that though the number of choices available has never been greater, rather than making people happier, it's leading to increased dissatisfaction. As he says: "Unfortunately, the proliferation of choice in our lives robs us of the opportunity to decide for ourselves just how important any given decision is."

Too much choice has a number of consequences, according to Barry. It fosters heightened expectations and, with it, decision regret. With so many options, trade-offs are inevitable. As he identifies, these have psychological consequences and "affect the level of satisfaction we experience from the decisions we ultimately make." Moreover, given the alternatives (the unselected choices), post-decision regret will almost always follow when a decision falls short of the desired result. Schwartz identifies an important cultural shift as a part of his analysis. Namely, that the decision-making onus increasingly falls on the individual—whether it's selecting healthcare insurance, college courses, or even an internet provider. The result is choice overload and the consequential fatigue reduces people's ability to make more difficult life decisions.

Defining goals

Given the cost of a bad decision, it's little wonder that outcome bias is so prevalent. This is when a decision is judged on its outcome, rather than the quality of the decision itself at the time it was made. The good news is that there are some simple solutions to help you overcome both.

Barry advises that a way to curb decision overload is to limit the number of choices you make. He suggests beginning with an audit of your recent choices, itemizing the time and energy invested, as well as the satisfaction experienced. He says that by understanding your choice exposure, it's easier to focus on what's important. "Choice

A PRACTICAL GUIDE TO DECISION-MAKING

- Limit your options to avoid choice overload and decision fatigue—Barry suggests that two is ideal.
- Adopt the principles of slow thinking and use your curiosity to explore fully the options, making sure that each is of equal value.
- Accept that there's no guarantee of a good outcome. Decision-making can reveal new insights into what you most value, including the impact on all aspects of your life.
- Write down your decisions, including the options considered, and your intentions and personal commitment to them.

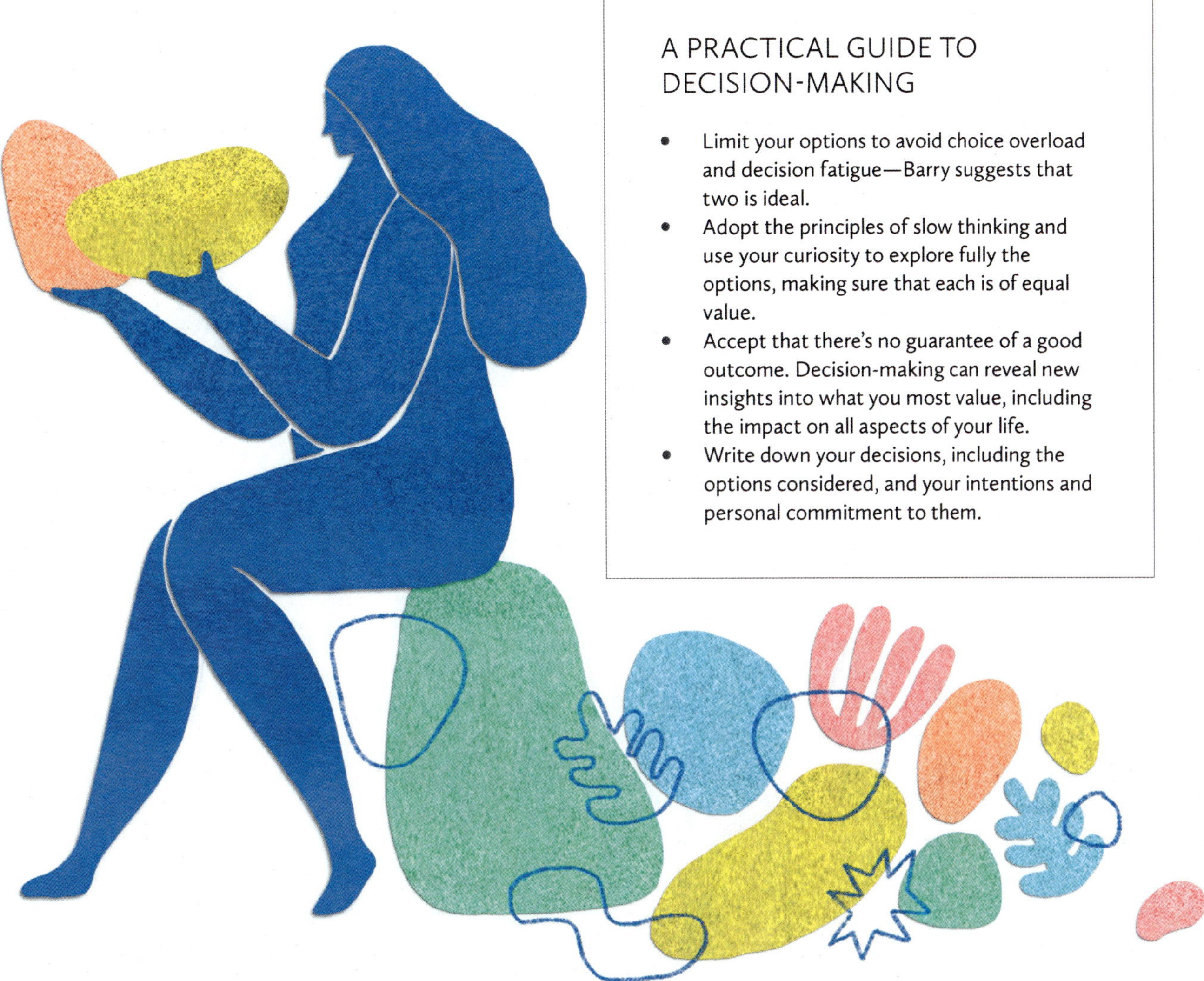

is what enables us to tell the world who we are and what we care about," he says. Moreover, he recommends focusing on the "good enough." By clearly defining your goals, each choice can be evaluated using personal criteria and standards. In doing so, you're what he calls a "satisficer"—your choice fulfills the minimum requirements of the goal—rather than a "maximizer," who, in pursuit of perfection, strives to make the choice that will give maximum benefit.

Accepting that it's almost impossible to predict the outcomes of decisions is also key, according to behavioral scientist Francesca Gino. She suggests greater importance should be given to the process of decision-making. In the podcast Choiceology, she says: "There's helpful information in both the intention and process that should really influence how we think about the quality of a decision."

Valuing ambiguity

One of the reasons people grapple with decisions is a dislike of ambiguity, preferring things to be more black and white. Weighing up the pros and cons is a technique frequently used to find the right decision, however, in reality, most options are rarely without benefits. This is why many people waiver between the alternatives, hoping that the best option will miraculously appear, or they simply don't make a decision at all. Rather than seeking the right decision, Oxford University professor Ruth Chang suggests viewing hard decisions as simply that. In *Hard Choices*, her paper for the *Journal of the American Philosophical Association*, she writes: "A choice can be hard because the alternatives are in the same neighborhood with respect to whatever matters in the choice, but neither is better than the other, nor are they equally good." She argues that difficult decisions occur because there's often no right answer—rather than their significance or a lack of information. It's for this reason that Chang suggests you personally commit to your decision, by creating a reason for investing in the option selected.

In our search for the right answer, it's often easy to overlook what is most valuable. Hard choices test who you are, and are opportunities for growth. All you need do is become more discerning about the decisions you make.

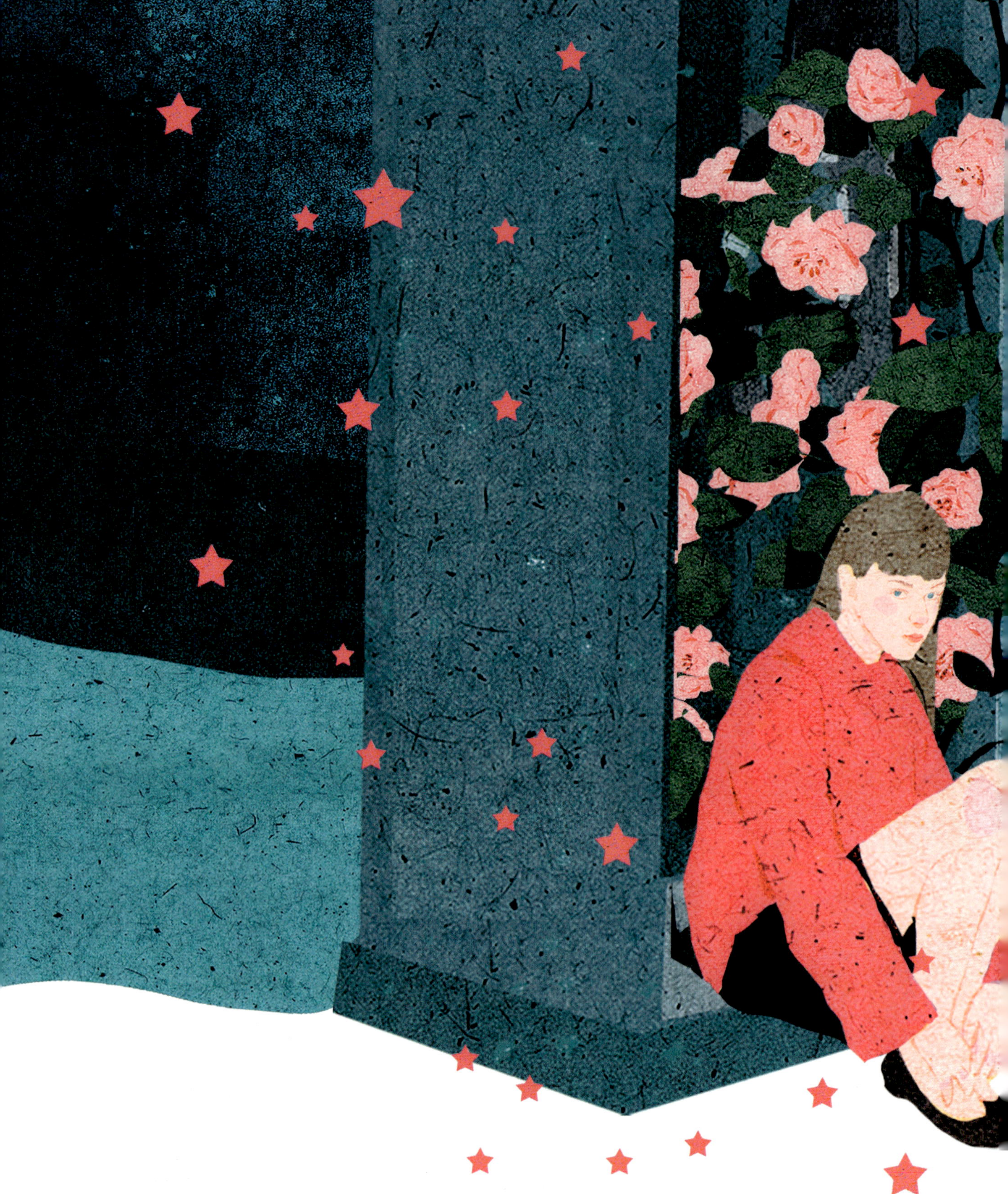

When dreams change

Do you have a childhood ambition or vision that remains unfulfilled? This isn't failure, but it might be an indication that your aspirations need an upgrade

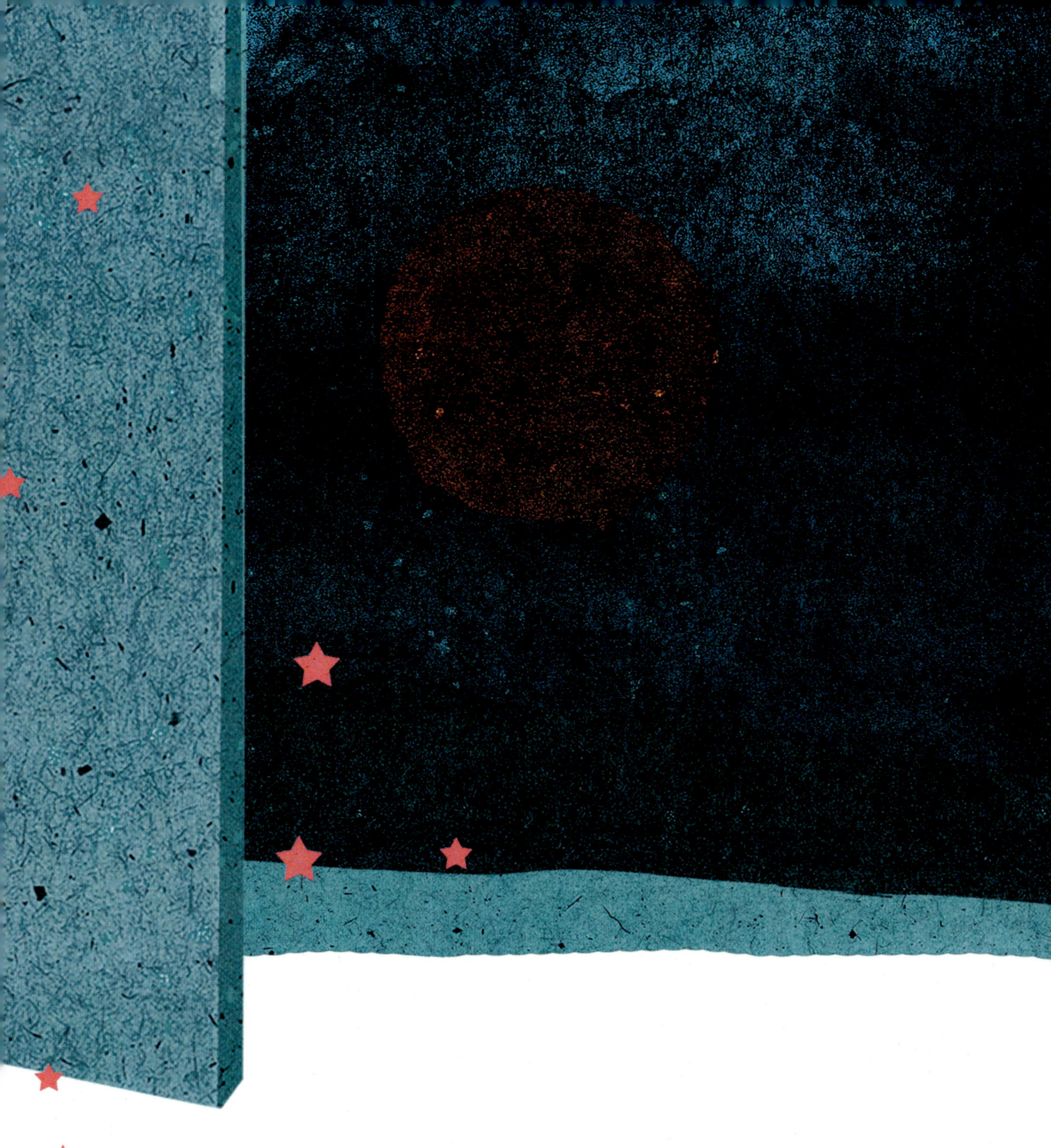

Ask a child what they want to be when they grow up and you'll often receive answers that foresee no limitations. From the days of those youthful dreams, negative experiences can erode confidence levels and unexpected hurdles or opportunities can shift priorities. As a result, many grown-ups find their childhood dreams, once so unwavering, go unrealized.

Such discussions usually elicit the response that "it's never too late." But in some instances, it's worth considering another possibility: perhaps it is too late to follow that particular dream. Perhaps, there was a good reason that it was never realized—one that had nothing to do with failure and far more to do with personal choice and a decision to follow a different path. And when traversing that path, you became a different person, with fresh passions. It might be that the dream your young self harbored is now outdated and ready for an upgrade because the thing about childhood dreams is they rarely keep up with your personal evolution. Through experiencing life, it's near impossible not to

"Throw your dreams into space like a kite, and you do not know what it will bring back, a new life, a new friend, a new love, a new country"

ANAÏS NIN

change. So why should goals you set as a seven-year-old remain the same? Sticking to what you think you know about yourself, rather than regularly checking in and reevaluating what you want, who you are, and what you've achieved, can stop you pursuing other opportunities. It can also leave you feeling like you've failed, which is not the case.

Learn to trust yourself

Rebecca Lockwood, award-winning mindset coach and founder of the Female Entrepreneurs Network, experienced postnatal depression. She was thrown off course but it was only then, when working through one of the hardest times in her life, that she discovered a new passion in an area where she hadn't been looking—in helping others to find their own purpose and freedom in the now.

"I had stopped sharing my childhood dreams by the time I became a mother," says Rebecca. "In my mind, I was a failure. Shortly after the birth of my first child I found myself sobbing, experiencing an empty feeling of not wanting to be here. It was then, in my darkest days, that I began studying NLP [neuro-linguistic programming, which is an approach to communication, personal development, and psychotherapy] and reevaluating my own life.

"It was through this that I was able to rediscover myself. I reevaluated my goals, my vision, my values. I checked back in with me and stopped trying to validate myself through others. I learned to trust myself. It was only then, with this newfound clarity, that I was able to determine what I really wanted out of life, in the present."

It's easy to get stuck perceiving yourself in the past. Weight or skin issues in younger years can be the cause of low self-esteem long after someone has physically transformed. Beliefs inherited from parents or others can also impair clarity if you don't give yourself the space to discover what's true for you. And goals set by your younger self, maybe before you even had a chance to figure out what really mattered to you, can hang around and feel important long after their validity has expired.

Rebecca believes that you never have to rule out your childhood goal—if you still want to achieve it. You might just need to take a new route. Before you do that, however, it's essential to check in with the present you. "Is this goal still something that you're passionate about?" asks Rebecca. "Or are you passionate about something else now you have evolved into a better, older, newer version?

"If you start reevaluating your goals based on these questions, you open up the chance to create a new, more empowering dream for yourself. And if it's the same or similar, that's okay too." Getting to know who you are today might reveal a different version to the one you've been imagining, as well as a fountain of new ambitions. But you must let yourself dream big, like you did as a child, so the aspirations flow from your heart as well as your head.

"As adults we sometimes shy away from our dreams. We no longer want to share with people that we long to perform on stage or fly a plane," says Rebecca.

"I've seen so many cases of self-sabotage, when we have underlying beliefs that we may not be aware of. Or imposter syndrome, which leads you to think you can't achieve this goal. Once you determine your new dream, don't question what you want, why you want it or how you're ever going to make it happen. Just trust that you will find a way and the universe will work in your favor."

Dream from a place of passion and joy

How do you find out whether or not childhood goals are still relevant to the present you? The key is personal alignment—a self-development concept (see right) that will help ensure the new goals you create, or the earlier ones you stick to, come only from a place of your innermost joy and passion, rather than as a means to make up for something you feel you lack, such as money, validation, or love.

Ask yourself if your goals, core values, and passions match up and if you're living in a way that allows you to experience and expand on these things. Real success, joy, and fulfillment is different for everyone, but it rarely comes down to the desire for wealth, status, or popularity on which many dreams are based. It doesn't come in the form of ticking off goals that you, or others, have set either. It comes from syncing up what you value most deeply, in the here and now, with the life that you are choosing to live.

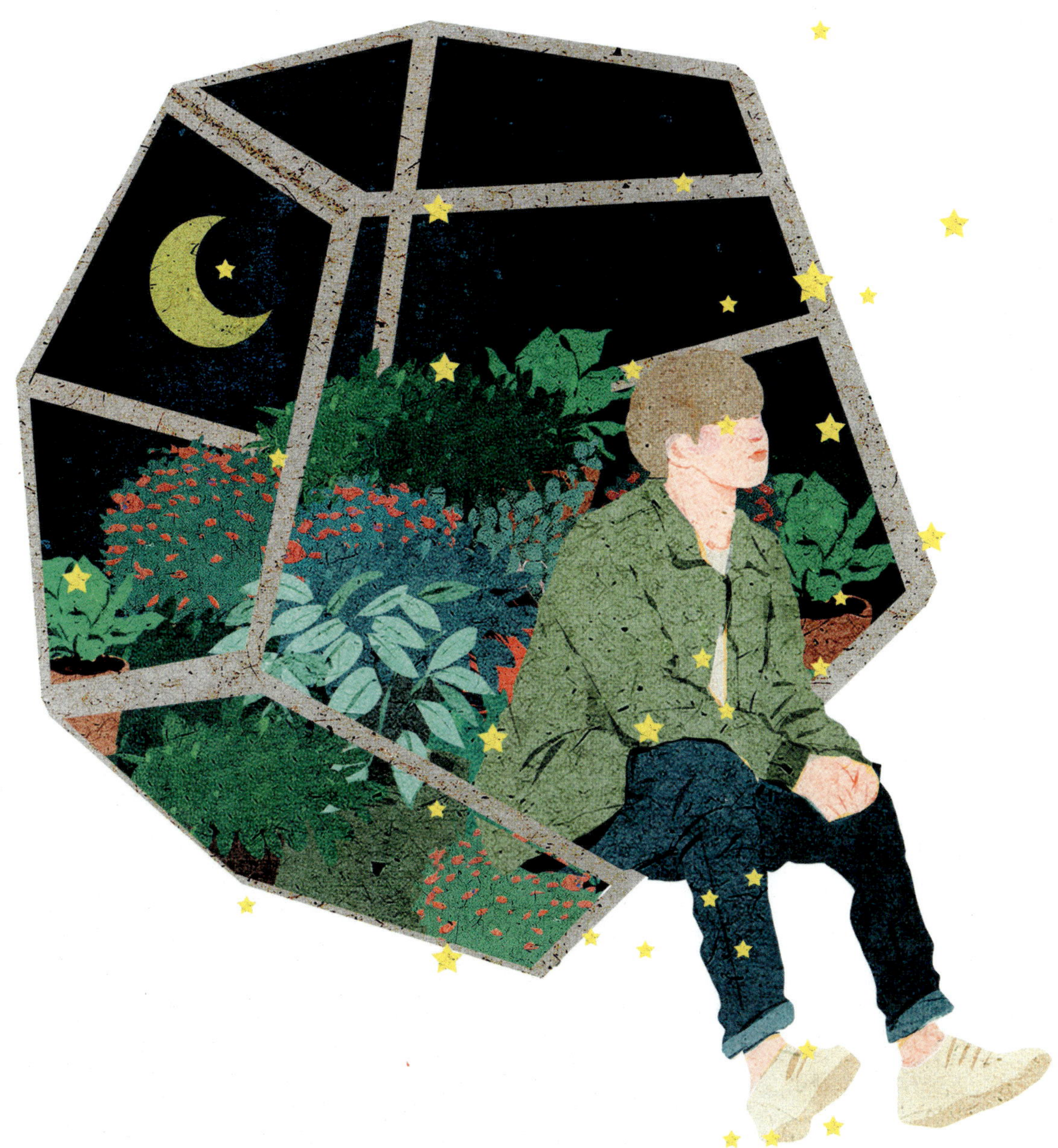

REEVALUATE YOUR LIFE GOALS

Practice personal alignment

Human beings are in a constant state of evolution, in many cases completely transforming, multiple times, through the years. And what lights you up is bound to change too. It's natural that goals set along the way might also evolve, so that they're in keeping with your most present self. The first step is figuring out who you are, right now, through personal alignment.

"Personal alignment is when you align yourself with what is important to you and begin to create a life based on that," explains Rebecca. "You can start with [something] as simple as placing your hand on your heart and asking 'Who am I?' and listening to what comes up."

What you discover might mean you have to shake things up to be able to live in alignment. This can be daunting, but be brave. It's incredibly rewarding.

Use stepping stones

Finding out that you have a new dream, or an old one you still wish to realize, is exciting. But it's not uncommon to feel stopped by the seemingly long road it could take to get there. Creating stepping stones to reach your long-term goal will help with this. If you're doing what you love, you'll enjoy and appreciate every success on your journey, not just the end result.

Rebecca recommends having overarching long-term goals and a newly written 90-day plan, every 90 days. This will give you momentum, satisfaction, progress, and the chance to check in with your ever-changing self, to see if you're still heading in the right direction.

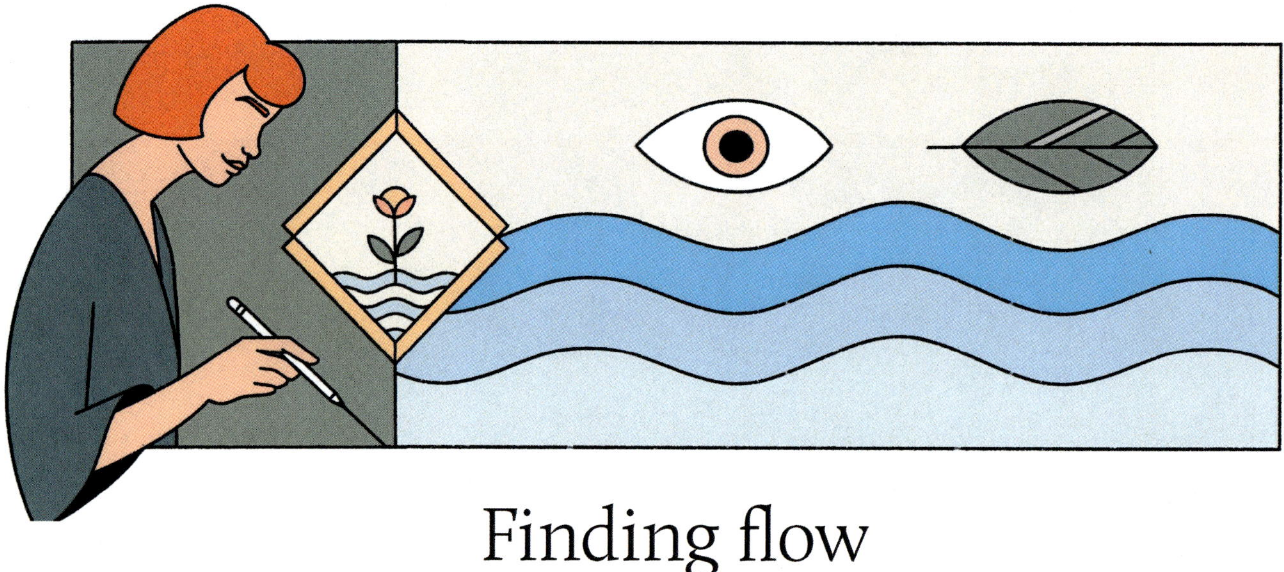

Finding flow

When you love what you're doing and you're doing it well, it's possible to achieve a higher state of mind

Imagine a place where it's possible to become so immersed in an activity that all sense of space and time is lost and physiological requirements, such as food, water, and sleep are deemed unimportant (if noticed). It's a place, or state of mind, that intrigued Hungarian psychologist, Mihály Csíkszentmihályi, who termed it "flow."

In the 1970s, Mihály, regarded as a founding father of the positive psychology movement, became fascinated by artists whose work was so all-consuming that they would enter this state. It was as if their activity became effortless, that their painting was somehow happening through them. In describing this state, several of the artists interviewed by Mihály used the metaphor of a current of water effortlessly carrying them along. Accordingly, the psychologist termed it the "flow state of mind."

The phenomenon wasn't confined to artists either. Musicians, athletes, martial-arts practitioners, and racing drivers entered a similar state, they just gave it a different name. For athletes it was "in the zone"; software developers talked of being "wired in"; stock-market traders were "in the pipe"; pool players called it "dead stroke."

Motivation and achievement

One way of thinking about flow is in terms of information processing. According to Mihály, a person typically processes around 110 bits of information each second. Decoding speech, for example, takes about 60 bits each second. This is why it's hard to focus on other things while conducting a conversation. In the flow state, all 110 bits of information are taken up by the activity. There's nothing left over. That's why people lose a sense of space and time and become oblivious to hunger, thirst, and sleep. The flow state is one of maximum motivation and maximum achievement. It's the human condition to face challenges and overcome them. This might be best done through breaking down the tasks into goals and applying requisite skills. In daily life, if people's skill levels are low and there's little to tax them, they might tend to feel apathy. When skill levels exceed challenges, there can be boredom whereas the converse can result in anxiety. When skills and challenges match, the person is achieving peak performance and likely to enter the flow state.

Intrinsic rewards

To achieve the flow state, motivation must be intrinsic—it comes from inside. Often, though, people are driven by extrinsic rewards, such as money, status, and sometimes fame. The greatest achievers tend to be most motivated by intrinsic reward—they want to do what they do. Money and fame are secondary. The flow state of seemingly effortless mastery, when people become lost in their performance, is most likely to happen when there's a love for the task or art. Perhaps a good example of intrinsic motivation is when mountaineer George Mallory was asked at a lecture why people wanted to climb Mount Everest. His reply was powerfully simple—"because it's there . . ." The human race is composed of problem solvers. Athletes, scientists, artists, and musicians are intent on solving problems, overcoming obstacles, and realizing opportunities in their respective disciplines. The greatest motivation will always be intrinsic—"because it's there . . ."

Mihály has postulated that people with a greater than average degree of intrinsic motivation are more likely to enter the flow state. Typically they also have high levels of curiosity and persistence. He termed them autotelic—from the Greek words autos (self) and telos (goal). Autotelic people are self-motivated and seek challenges to facilitate personal growth.

Flow can also be a group phenomenon. Throughout history, people have banded together to face challenges—a Stone Age hunting party is a classic example. It's human nature to cooperate with others. Musicians jamming together might suddenly find themselves in a state of flow and so may an orchestra, whose members surprisingly find themselves giving the performance of their lives. But flow can occur in any activity.

The world of work comprises a major proportion of most people's lives. In his book, *Good Business: Leadership, Flow, and the Making of Meaning*, Mihály examined working life. A fundamental principle of management is the need to provide an environment for people to toil in a purposeful, effective, and fulfilling manner. In 1968, the American psychologist Fred Herzberg published a study, *One More Time: How Do You Motivate Employees?* Its ideas dovetail with those of Mihály.

Fred made a crucial distinction between what he termed hygiene factors, such as salary and working conditions, and what he termed motivational factors, including job satisfaction and personal growth. It's important to provide the former but beyond a certain point, they'll no longer galvanize people. It's getting the motivational factors right that opens the door to peak performance. Here, hygiene factors are extrinsic, whereas motivational factors are intrinsic. Doing something because you love it is intrinsic, and people doing what they love will tend to outperform those who aren't doing what they love—and they'll be far more likely to achieve a state of flow. When managers achieve optimum hygiene and motivational factors performance can soar—at an individual level, at a team level, and at an overall level—delivering huge benefits to employees and clients. They can transform people's lives.

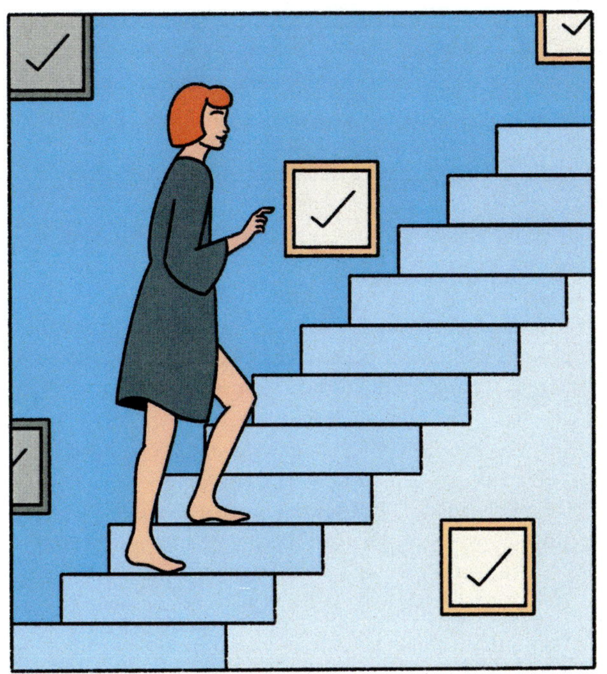

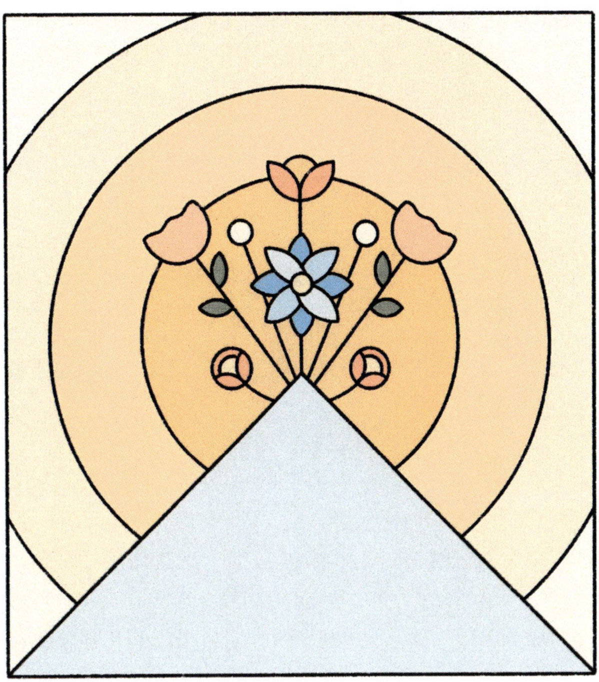

Mihály also distinguished between pleasure and enjoyment. Pleasure is passive (for example, eating an ice cream) whereas enjoyment is active (playing a game to the best of one's ability). Pleasure is transitory and easily forgotten, whereas enjoyment is deeper and more fulfilling because people are investing much more of themselves. The more fulfilling the pursuit, the more likely it is that a participant will experience the flow state.

Setting goals

The simplest way to achieve flow is to get into the habit of goal-setting. There's abundant evidence from myriad disciplines, including athletics and business, that successful people are goal-setters. For some, this seems to come naturally but for others it's learned. Ultimately, achieving goals—or milestones—is the route to success.

The notion of goal-setting implies challenge, pushing yourself, and personal growth. Each achieved goal is both a reward in itself and the precursor to the next target, which will often be more challenging and may require an increase in skill level. When goals are clear-cut and precise, when they're at the limit of a person's skill level and, crucially, where there's immediate feedback (think of a racing driver, constantly making adjustments), then it's much more likely that the flow state of peak performance will occur.

It's no coincidence that two of Mihály books are entitled *Flow: The Psychology of Optimal Experience* and *Flow: The Psychology of Happiness*. For him, happiness is not about extrinsic rewards such as money or kudos. It's intrinsic, it's a state of mind. It's about doing what you love and loving what you do. And when you do it best—when you achieve peak performance—it will feel delightfully effortless. You'll be like a leaf on the river, being carried along by the flow.

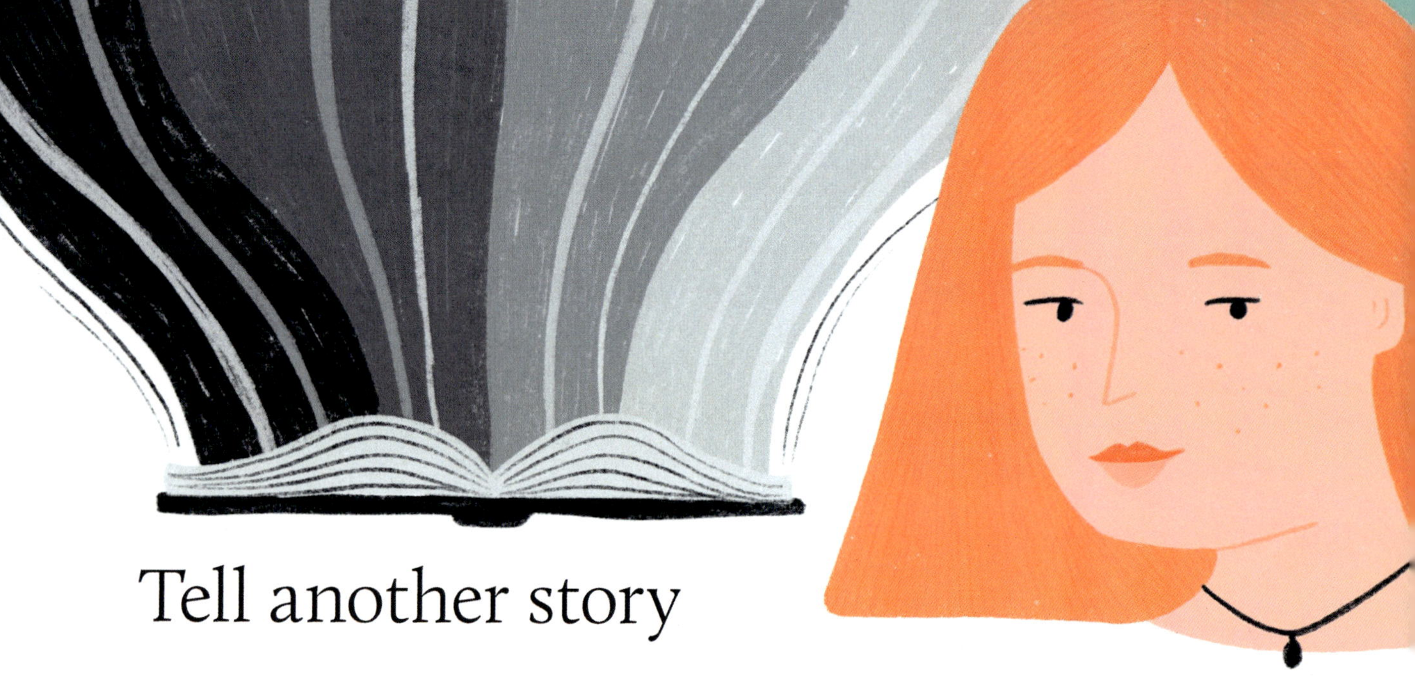

Tell another story

Is there one tale or belief you keep telling yourself that limits or holds you back? Is there a chance that it isn't actually true? Here's how to challenge it, as you might a person who continually undermines you, and replace it with a positive narrative that respects your ability

Raised on stories

"Everyone is brought up on stories," says Karen Kwong, a psychologist and founder of London-based Ren Organisational Consulting. "As you grow up, you subconsciously choose which of these to retain and then apply to the way you perceive yourself and others." It's these childhood narratives that shape the filters you use to view the world around you. This is, however, a form of survival, suggests Karen.

"You take in thousands of pieces of data every second. In order not to overload the brain, you've trained yourself to filter it. You make snap judgments about what's worth keeping and what isn't." These assessments illustrate the way filters are shaped by upbringing. A person might, for instance, have grown up in a deeply conservative household and look at life in a very structured way. "Even if you end up rebelling and shunning the conservatism, it's still a reaction to your childhood experience," says Karen. "You've simply gone from one extreme to the other."

Survival instinct

The human brain's negativity bias is well documented by scientists. Humans habitually hang on to or seek out negative thoughts and shun the opposite—it's an instinctual response to life. These narratives are a built-in survival mechanism that allow you to assess what could go wrong. "It's a physiological fight-or-flight response," explains Karen. "You're taught from an early age to look out for threats, and your primary filters help you survive."

What's more, this bias becomes evident in many situations. "If someone pays you a compliment," says Karen, "you may thank them initially then quickly look for a caveat to counteract the compliment, such as having bad hair or feeling fat."

It can also seem just as natural to focus on your own negative interpretation of an event—perhaps ruminating on it for days. "Whatever else happened at the time, you may remember just one thing, such as something you said that you wish you hadn't. Meanwhile, everyone else will remember the event differently, according to their own values, beliefs, and filters."

Back to school

Natalie Costa is a life coach and founder of Power Thoughts, a practice that supports children as young as five through the experience of growing up. Essentially, she helps them to challenge their negative beliefs—something she calls "unwanted visitors." Natalie explains: "At school you're taught to think critically and to solve problems, but you're not necessarily taught about the power of those thoughts or your ability to choose them."

Natalie teaches her students that they don't have to believe every thought that pops into their head. "Most of their fears are very similar to adult fears. Worrying about raising your hand in class in case people laugh at you feels the same as speaking up in a meeting. Being nervous about attending a party evokes the same nerves as networking in a room of strangers. This is the time of life, from age five, that children's beliefs begin to form—including any limiting beliefs."

It is, however, never too late to change these thoughts. Age is irrelevant. "Fear and excitement may be two very different emotions, but they can generate the same feelings in the body. You can flip the fear by telling your brain that you're excited instead. For example: 'I'm excited to give this presentation or take this exam because I've rehearsed or prepared for it so much.' It can help you to focus on the positive."

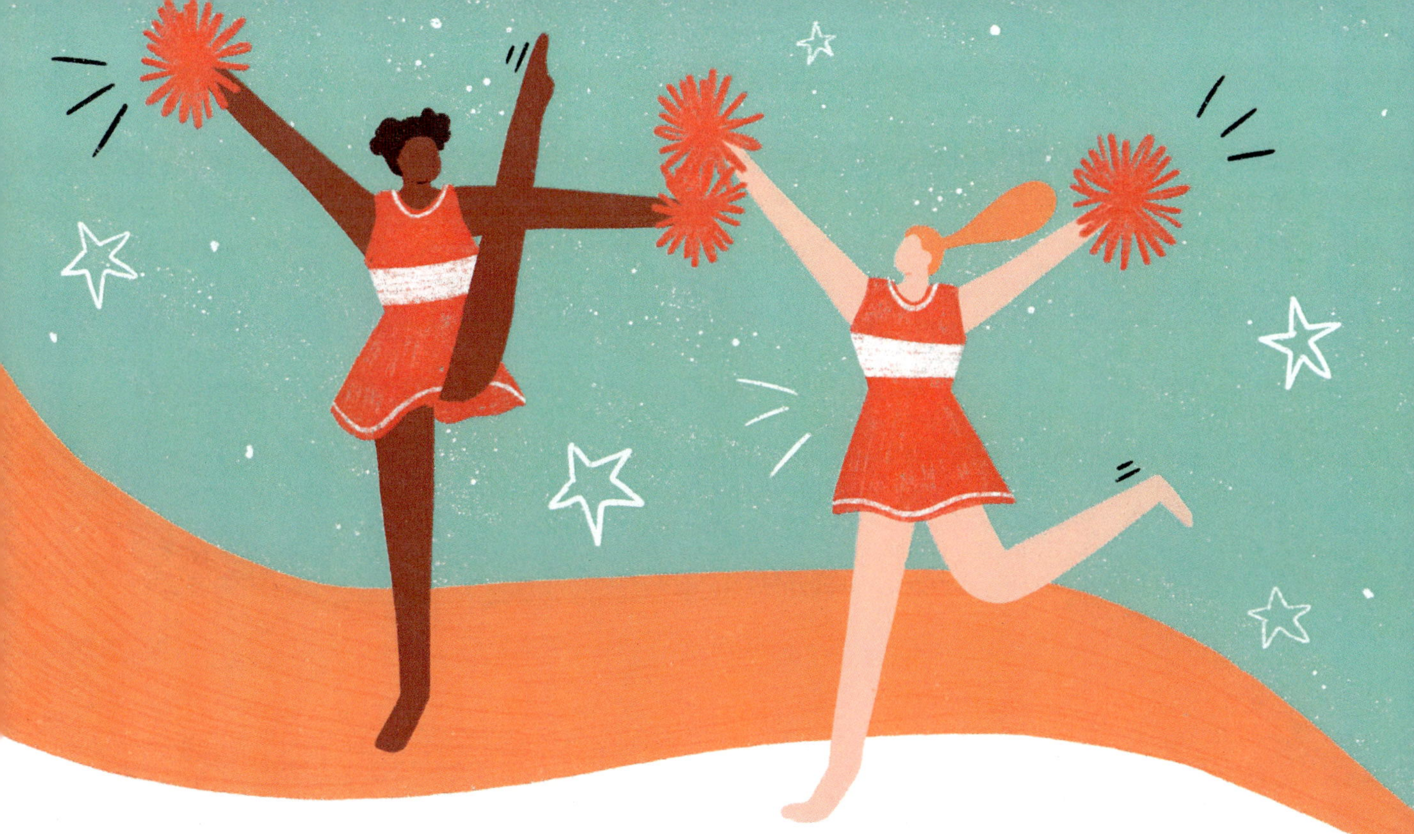

Rubber banding

Don't be alarmed if focusing on positive thoughts makes you feel uncomfortable. The fight-or-flight programming has been running since childhood, so the neural pathways that seek danger run deep. They feel safer and less challenging than the unknown territory of more affirmative beliefs.

While you're practicing the new stories, it's possible that you will "rubber band" or bounce back and forth between the known and the unknown. This is a perfectly natural process. Eventually the rubber will weaken and snap as you carve new neural pathways, making it easier and more comfortable to cultivate happier thoughts.

Train your brain

In so far as the negative narrative may have become normal, so can the positive. You can train your brain to form new ideas and stories. "It's all about working the part that hasn't been used as often," says Karen, "just as you'd train a different muscle in a gym, or you'd try some yoga if you'd been running for a long time." Your body tells you what you need, but your mind doesn't. This is where mindfulness comes in useful.

"Most people don't hear themselves, or don't take time to think about what they're thinking. So mindfulness isn't about clearing your mind, but checking in with it, and observing what's going for you right now," says Karen. "You could set an alarm every hour to remind yourself to stop and listen to your thoughts and feelings. Write them down and look back at what you've written after one week—would you speak to a friend in the same way?"

Listen without becoming attached to certain thoughts or feelings, or habitually obsessing about how bad they are. "When you feel anxious and you tell yourself, 'I am anxious,' the anxiety can consume or become you," adds Karen. "Yet if you acknowledge that the anxiety will eventually go away, this creates a degree of separation." The anxiety—or any other uncomfortable feeling—is not who you are. It's how you feel in a particular moment. You might even see it as a visitor who's just popping in for a while but will soon leave.

Welcome the visitors

If these visitors are unwelcome, as Natalie teaches, you can give them a personality, a voice, and a name—create a caricature that mocks them a little and removes the power you believe this visitor holds over you. This exercise can help to remind you that you're in charge of your thoughts. Try this with the limiting belief or story that crops up most often. Hold the image of the visitor in your mind and ask them the following questions:

What unhelpful things do you say to me?
How do you make me feel?
Who could I be without you?

This is a tool that Natalie encourages both children and adults to use. "Let your inner child come out to play since the fears you had when you were younger may be similar to the ones you have now. If you personify these thoughts, you know it's not you, but just another voice. This means you can also create other voices, like a positive character, a best friend, or cheerleader who supports you."

Getting into the habit of challenging your negative beliefs on a regular basis can help you to replace them with more positive ones. Try recording them for a week using the exercise on the following page.

FIND THE FICTION

It's not always easy to supplant a damaging narrative with something kinder and more compassionate, but it's hugely beneficial to do so since negative thoughts can cause stress, anger, frustration, and sadness. If your limiting beliefs are lingering, then challenge them. Once you begin to question them, they will lose their power over you. Begin by writing the thought down on paper then ask yourself the following:

Is it true?

....

....

....

....

....

....

....

What evidence do I have?

....

....

....

....

....

....

....

How is this helpful to me?

....

....

....

....

....

....

....

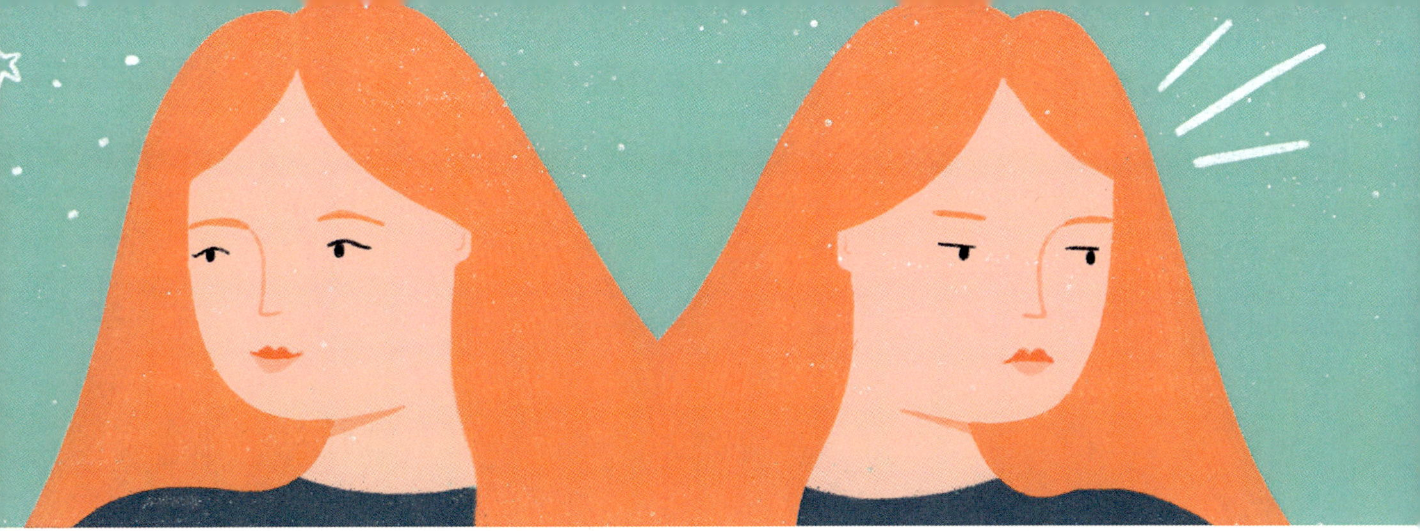

How does it make me feel?

How would I feel if the opposite were true?

Who could I be without this thought?

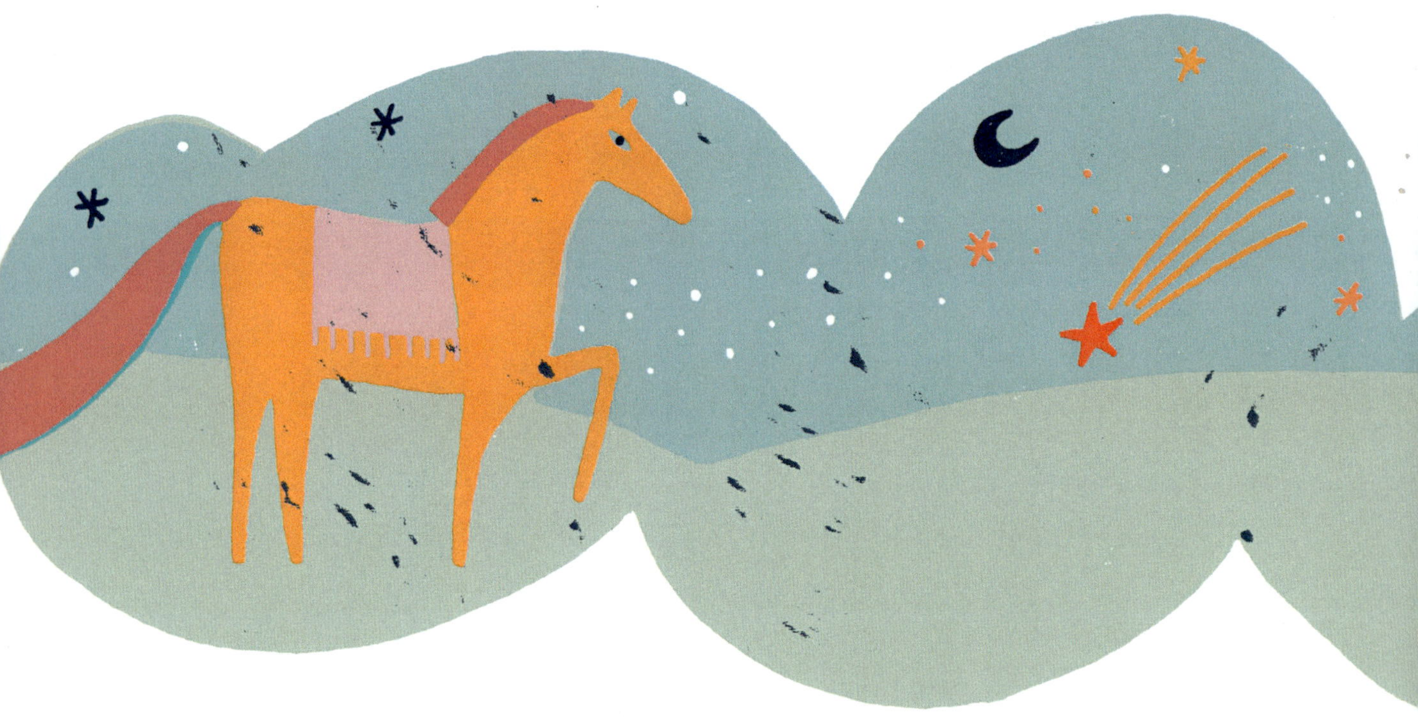

Character building

Reading out loud is often abandoned once childhood is over. But re-embracing your inner storyteller is an old-fashioned form of self-care that can help to bridge the generation gap, alleviate loneliness, and open up a whole new vocabulary

Apparently, master story writer Roald Dahl loved to read aloud his scary tales to his enthralled family while in a dark, damp, railway tunnel. The combination of the words and location would have certainly helped ramp up the spook factor, but as research is increasingly finding, reading out loud has powerful benefits—not just for the listener, but for the storyteller, too.

Who doesn't remember the sheer joy of being read to as a child? A kind of magic happens when someone narrates a story—the words spring to life, coalescing into a powerful fuel for the heart, brain, and imagination. If you're a parent, there's a good chance you carried on this age-old tradition with your own children, perhaps as part of the bedtime routine or, as they got older, to help with their studies.

For anyone with younger people in the picture, be they grandchildren, godchildren, nieces and nephews, or friends' and neighbors' offspring, there are compelling reasons to dust off those books (or grab a Kindle) once more. Meghan Cox Gurdon, a children's literature reviewer for *The Wall Street Journal*, shared her passion for the benefits of reading out loud in her book, *The Enchanted Hour: the Miraculous Power of Reading Aloud in The Age of Distraction.*

"Like a lot of people, I always had the general idea that it was something meaningful and lovely and deeply cozy," she says. "But then I did it with my children and it felt like something real. It was the gift of time and of a voice. The telling of stories is a source of pleasure that has been available to human beings of all ages since before the printed word."

She has a point—it's something the ancient Greeks believed in, too. They thought it strange to read to oneself, rather than sharing the words with an audience.

An interlude in daily life

Meghan, who is a mother of five, still devotes time each evening to narrating to her offspring, some of whom are nudging their 20s. First off the book shelf is often the Robert Louis Stevenson classic, *Treasure Island*—a thrilling tale about Jim Hawkins' boyhood quest for buried riches.

"There is a lot going on, sentence to sentence. It is quite sophisticated language, with lots of personalities, and that is more fun to read aloud," she says of her choice. "It's [also] exciting, there is action. I do prefer reading classics to older kids, because there seems invariably to be so much more going on in the writing, with the language, than in many contemporary books."

Meghan touches on the emotional and intuitive benefits of reading out loud, remarking on how it provides a lovely interlude in daily life where you wrap children

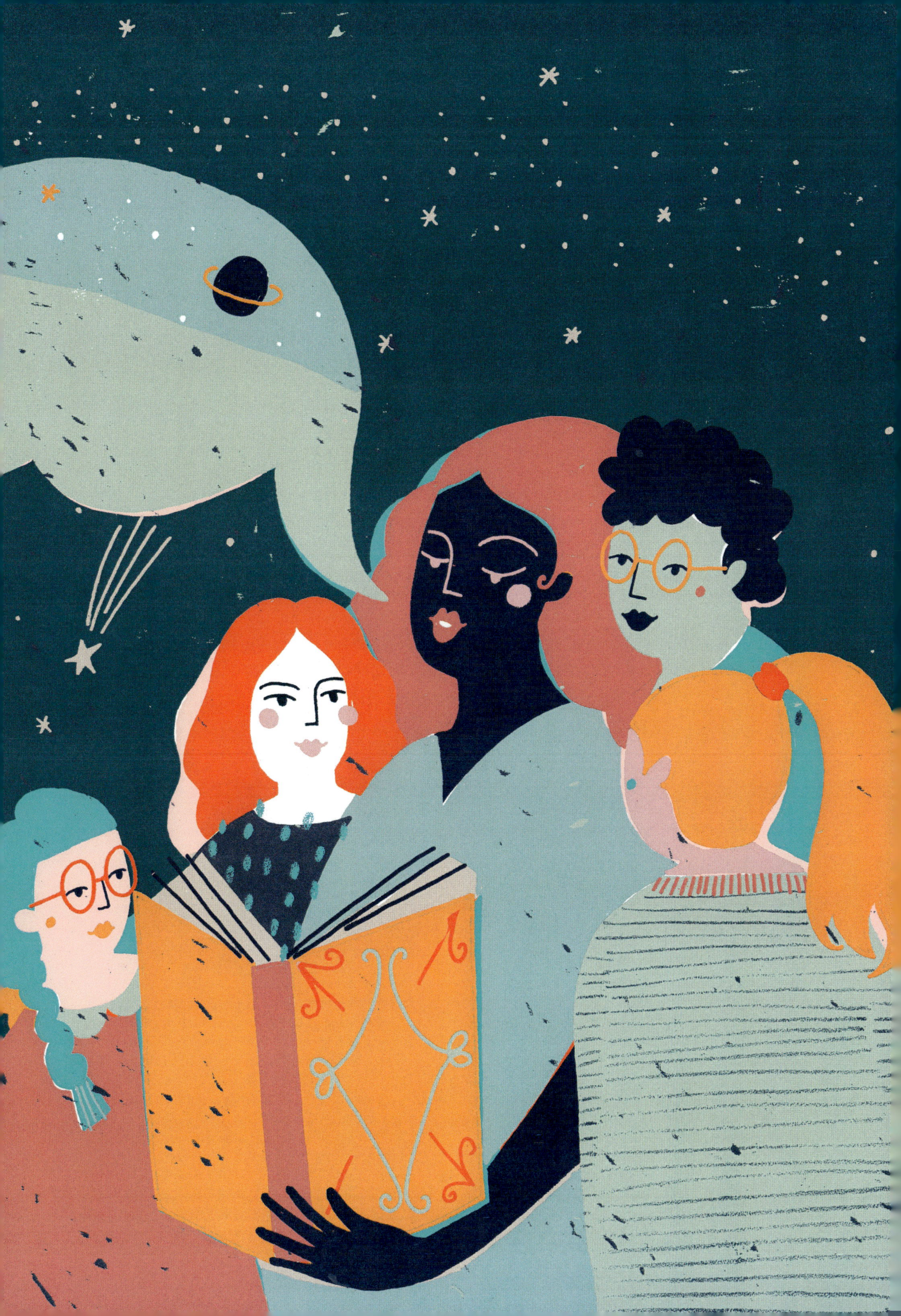

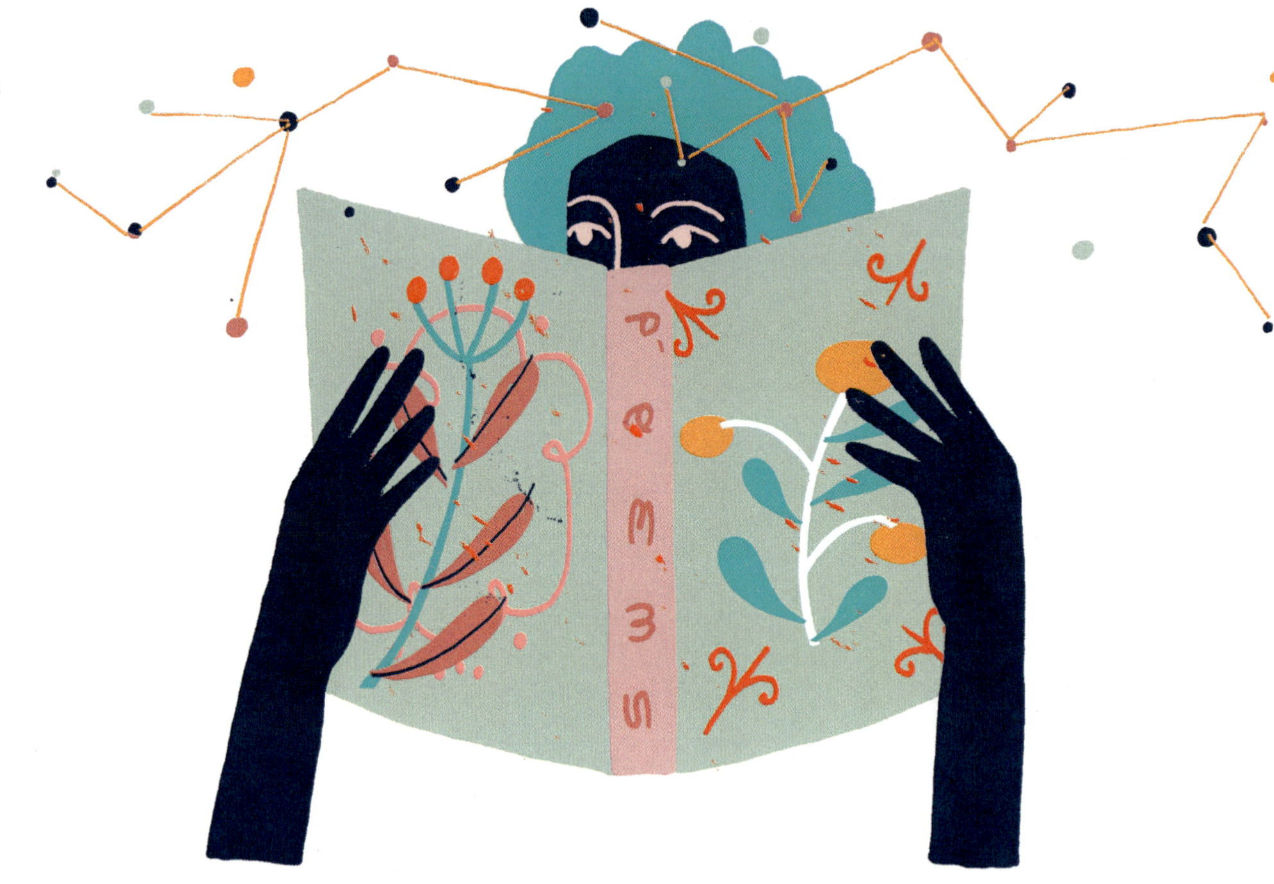

"So please, oh please, we beg, we pray, go throw your TV set away, and in its place you can install a lovely bookshelf on the wall"

ROALD DAHL

in a circle of warmth and it strengthens family and friendship bonds. It's a time when you accompany them into the realm of the imagination, while boosting their vocabularies and encouraging empathy, enabling them to relate to their own life experiences and solve problems. Along the way, hopefully, they'll also inherit the gift of reading for pleasure.

Charity and champion of the power of books, World Book Day, has tapped into the importance of reading out loud with its #ShareAStory campaign, which encourages parents, carers, siblings, and friends to read to one another for at least 10 minutes a day. This also encourages people of every age to put down their digital devices, something with which Meghan is fully on board. "Many people are thirsting for the love and meaning and connection that reading aloud offers, not only out of nostalgia, but also because it offers an antidote to the ill-defined, tech-associated ennui that ails so many of us."

While it's near impossible to measure the intangible benefits of reading out loud, scientific research highlights cognitive benefits, especially for older people. First up, researchers at the University of Waterloo discovered a phenomenon they call the "production effect." In short, their experiments found that reading aloud made words easier to remember than when they were only read silently. Verbally pronouncing a word creates a memorable experience, while the brainpower used to encode the word in speech helps to bank it in the long-term memory. This will be welcome news to people of a certain age who have noticed a slower—and maddening—process of word recall.

Warren Buffett, the business magnate, is referred to as the Wizard of Omaha because he's regarded as one of the greatest investors who ever lived. He created his billionaire and third-richest-man-in-the-world status through a shrewd understanding of the stock market.

Warren says that he spends around 80 percent of his day reading. Whether that's aloud or silent, at a not-so-sprightly 90, he is pretty persuasive proof that reading in older age may well be one of the secrets to preserving mental ability. Taking this one exciting step further are researchers at University of Liverpool in the UK. They've suggested that reading poetry aloud can help people living with dementia by stimulating the brain's neural pathways. So, it seems that reading aloud might also help to keep any creaky cogs moving.

Canadian Stephanie Ciccarelli, cofounder of Voices.com, a website for voiceover artists, talks about the focus aspect of giving voice to words. "When you're reading aloud, you will find that it becomes easier to put all of your energy into the task at hand without the temptation of distractions," she says. "You are so focused that you likely won't even notice you are strengthening your mental and verbal skills. If you think about it, your mind is akin to a muscle. When it works out, you tone it and build up strength. When you read aloud, you are exercising the connection between your mind and your voice to the full extent, which results in greater focus and cohesiveness."

But beyond the brain-kindling effects of reading out loud, there are other soul-enriching side-effects. It can be huge fun, especially if you create different voices for different characters. The sillier you are, the quicker you'll be able to access your own inner child, too. Also, if you pick new authors, it offers a pleasurable lesson in an ever-evolving language. There's a good chance the child you're reading to will become your teacher, explaining new words and phrases that crop up.

Also, by creating a relaxed, intimate space, children may be encouraged to open up about anything that may be on their mind while older people might find that any feelings of loneliness are lessened. This pull toward a natural sharing of concerns is especially true for both adults and teens with a welcome means of communication, without the nagging, negativity, and silences that often creep into that dynamic. As Stephanie says: "It is a wonderful way of being together without having that pressure or being asked lots of questions." And the best news about getting your own storyteller on? Dark, damp railway tunnels are purely optional.

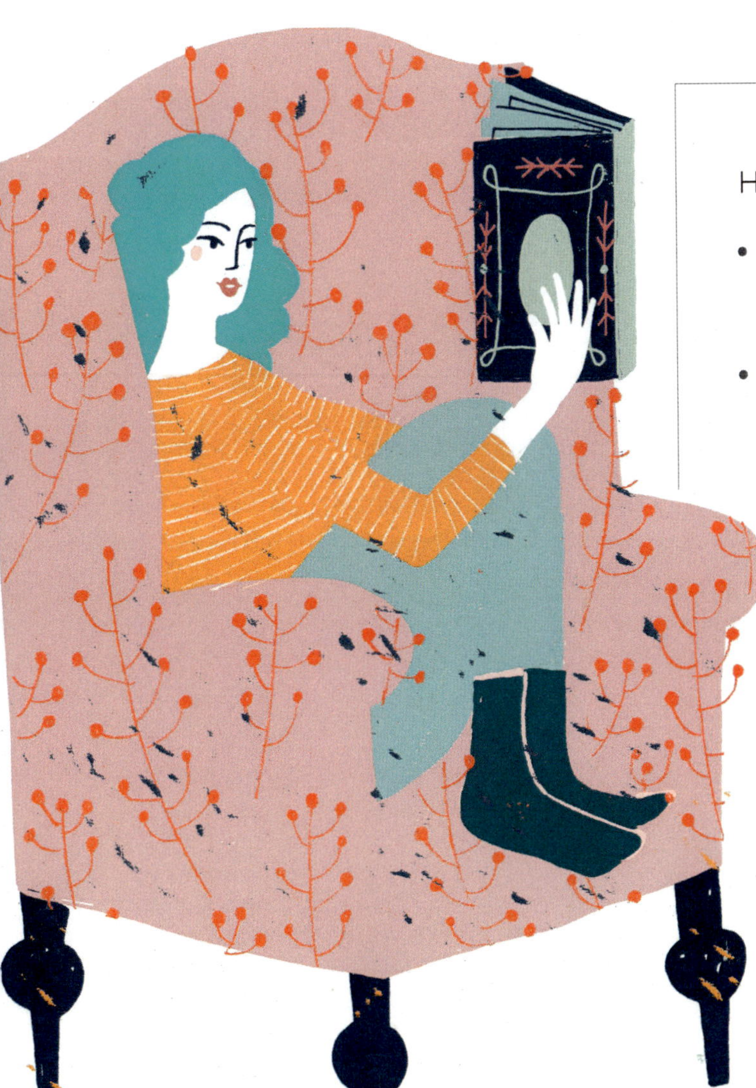

HOW TO SPIN A GOOD YARN

- Skim-read the book ahead of your storytelling session so you have an idea of the main themes and characters.
- Props can help add an extra layer to the story and are especially useful if the children are fidgety. They don't have to be elaborate: Roald Dahl used a bamboo cane as a stand-in for the trumpet of one of his most-beloved creations, the BFG.

C.S. Lewis said: "Since it is so likely that they will meet cruel enemies, let [children] at least have heard of brave knights and heroic courage. Otherwise you are making their destiny not brighter but darker." The Lewis classic, *The Chronicles of Narnia*, contains all of these magical themes—main character Aslan the lion is the embodiment of goodness and justice—and the book is sure to be a winner.

The Boy in the Dress by David Walliams, *The Phoenix and the Carpet* by E. Nesbit, and *The Wizard of Oz* by L. Frank Baum are all great books to get you started.

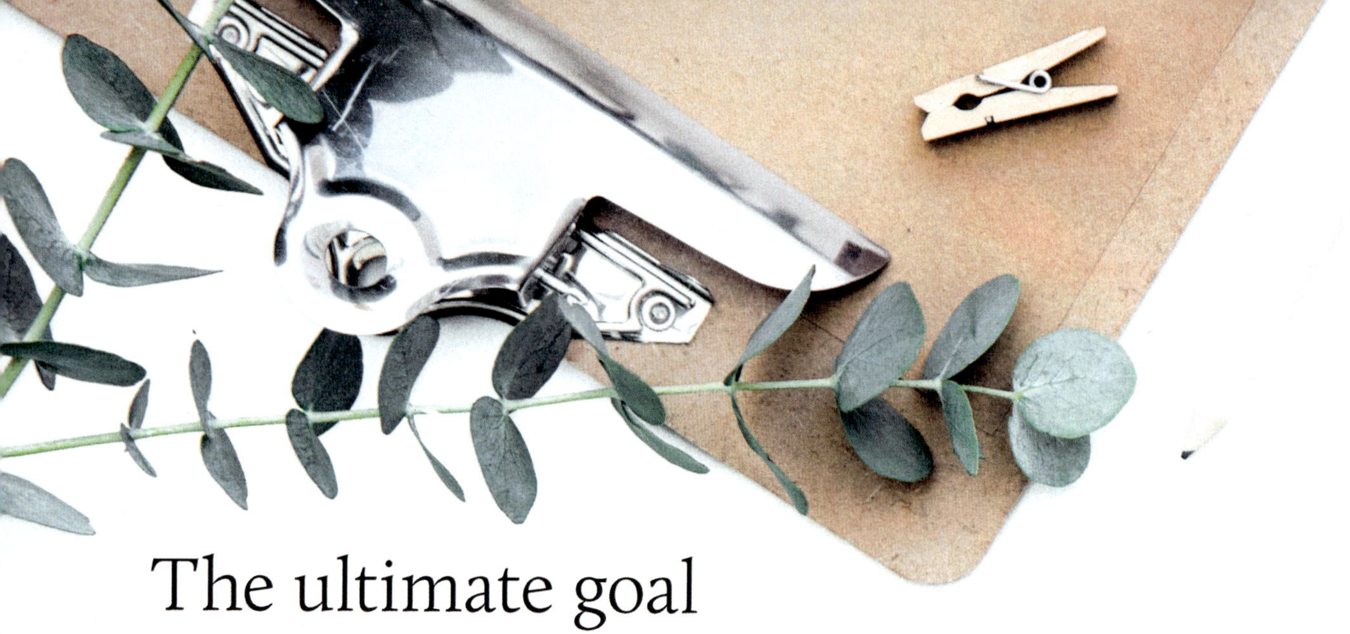

The ultimate goal

Visualizing your best future and capturing it on paper can help to make dreams a reality

How would you like your life to be in one, five, or 10 years? Do you find yourself daydreaming about future success or are you more consumed by future anxieties? Journaling is not just a powerful way to process your feelings in the present, but it can even help you to create the future of your dreams. Research has found that writing about your best possible future self can help to improve your happiness, but can it also make your dreams and goals become a reality? Possibly. A study by psychology professor Gail Matthews at Dominican University of California discovered that those who wrote down their goals accomplished more than those who didn't.

Many athletes use visualization techniques to improve their performance. They see themselves crossing the finish line, and create a vivid scene using all the senses. They hear the roar of the crowd and the feel of their feet on the running track.

The principle of imagining or dreaming about your future may subtly affect your thinking in ways you may not consciously be aware of and help your dreams become a reality. In one research study, people interacted with their future self via a virtual reality game. Researchers found that those people were more likely to put money into an experiment-based retirement account than those that didn't interact with their future self.

Writing is a great way to ruminate on your future self as well as letting go of the anxieties that can get in the way of reaching your goals. Here are a few exercises to try . . .

How do you feel about the future?

Do you have dreams that feel hard to reach? Are you filled with fear about what might go wrong? What thoughts come to you when you consider your future? Write it all down without censoring yourself, even the thoughts that feel negative or scary. You might like to take around 10 to 15 minutes to do this to clear your mind before going onto the next stage. Destroying the writing afterward, or throwing it in the trash, can be a symbolic way to let go of anything you don't want.

Your best possible future self

Take 20 to 30 minutes (or longer) to imagine your best possible future self. Visualize yourself and use all of the five senses in your description. You could answer the questions below, and anything else that brings the scene to life:

- What do you have with you?
- What is your job?
- Where do you live?
- What do you do for fun?
- What are the personality strengths or character traits that will help you reach your goals?

Listen to your mind

Has completing these exercises helped you feel more positive about the future? Do you find yourself thinking of new ideas or establishing new goals that will make your dreams a reality? In the days after completing the exercise, notice how it may have affected your thinking. You might find that instead of falling back on old habits like "I can't" or "it's not possible for me," you may create a little mental space that opens up the possibility that your desired future can become a reality.

As you go about your daily life, be mindful of your thoughts. If you find yourself sliding back into negative thinking, then pick up your pen and repeat these exercises. Writing about your future self is a journaling exercise that you can return to again and again. It can help to shift your mindset if you're feeling low or when you hit an emotional wall and think that your goals are just too far out of reach.

You can do it for the long or short term. For example, you could visualize yourself doing well in a job interview or succeeding at a networking event. The future begins with your thoughts. All you need do is pick up your pen.

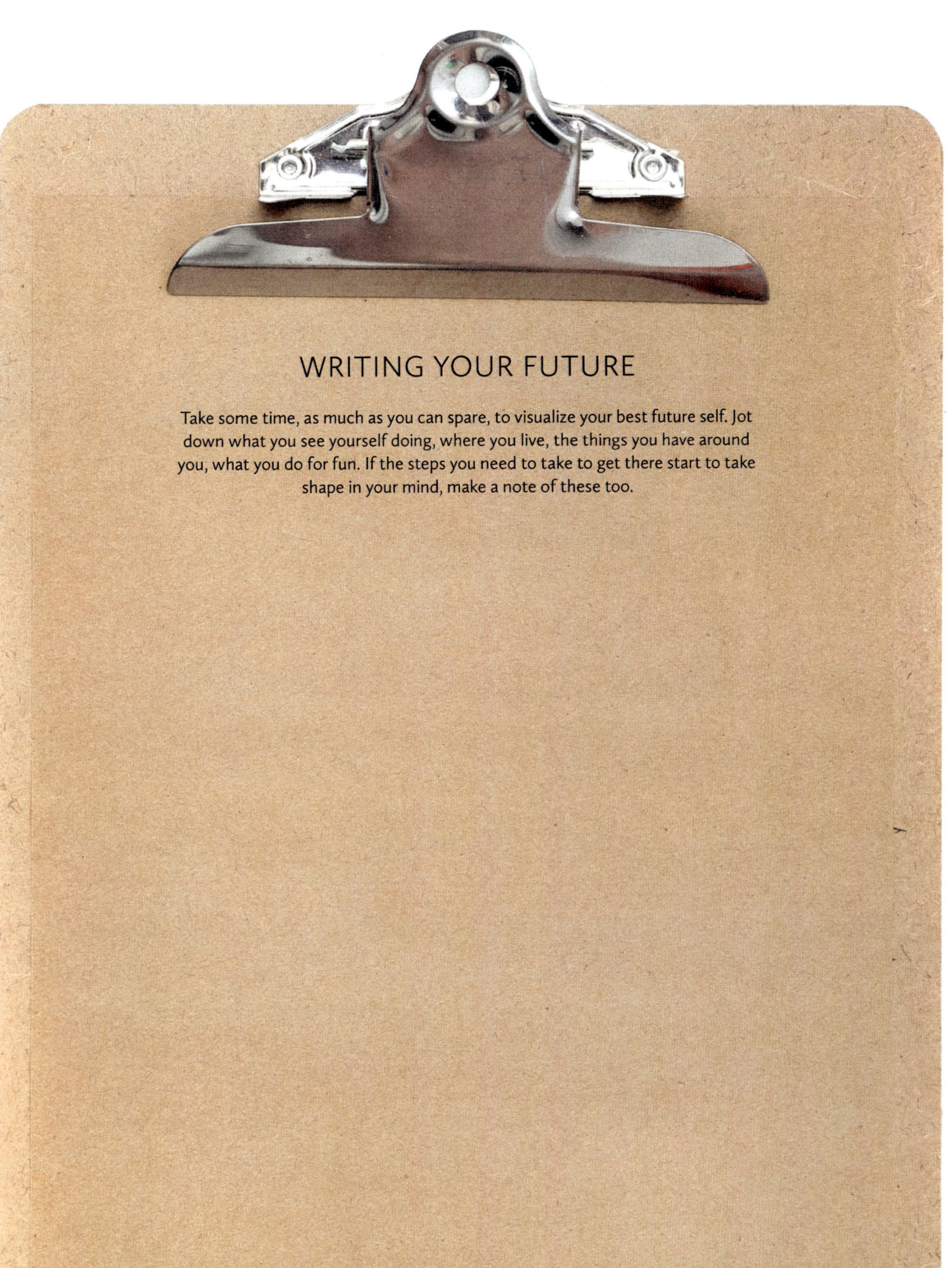

WRITING YOUR FUTURE

Take some time, as much as you can spare, to visualize your best future self. Jot down what you see yourself doing, where you live, the things you have around you, what you do for fun. If the steps you need to take to get there start to take shape in your mind, make a note of these too.

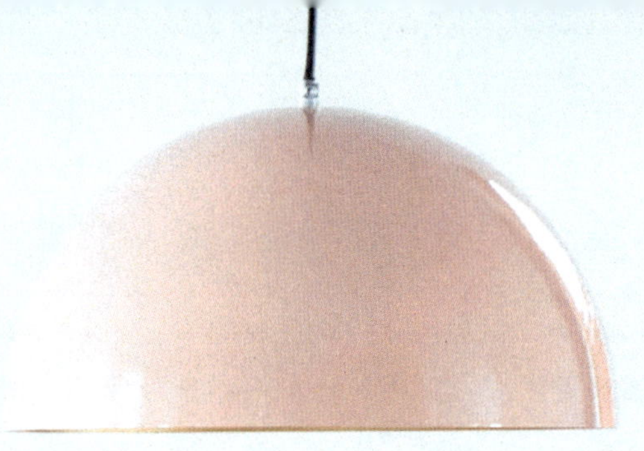

Wonder walls

A lick of paint, a new rug on the floor, a desk by the window—discover ways to improve your well-being wherever you work or dwell

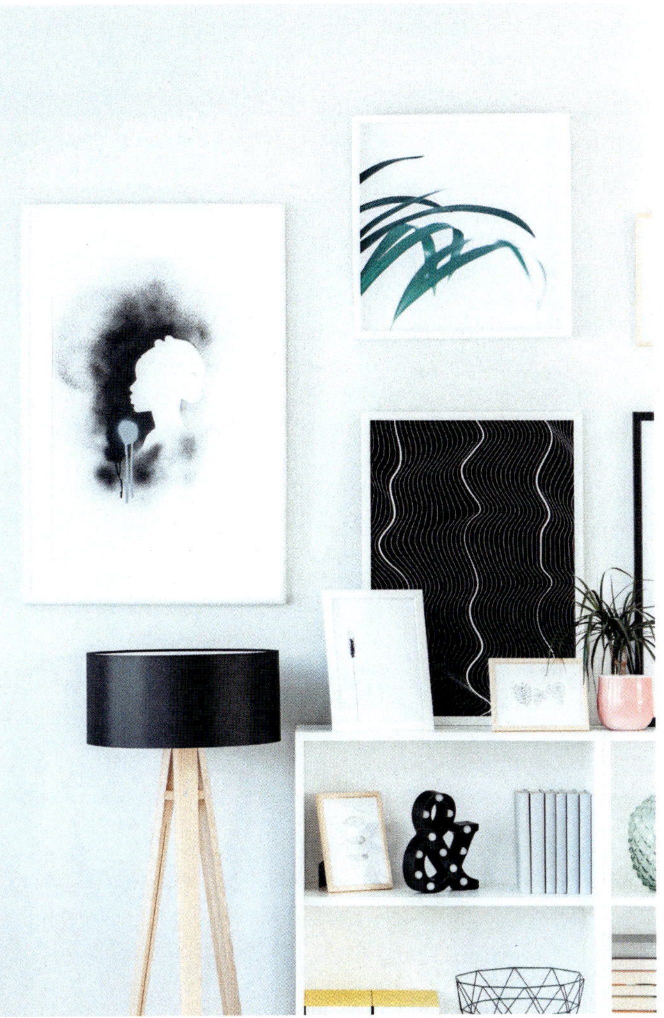

Anyone who's played the video game The Sims will know that when you hang a painting on the wall, your Sim's Mood goes up. As a teenager, I never thought this was realistic—the idea that a person's state of mind could drastically increase because of an object. The truth is, though, your surroundings play a huge role in the way you think and feel. While your mood boost (or decline) might not be as immediate as in The Sims, studies now suggest that how beautiful your immediate environment looks can make a big difference to well-being, with benefits to overall health.

For some, one way to make a space feel beautiful is to keep it clutter-free. No matter how nicely decorated a house or office is, if it's untidy, it tends to detract from the aesthetics. Cluttered spaces can also have negative consequences for well-being. A US study by Darby Saxbe and Rena Repetti found people living in messy homes had far slower rates of decline of the hormone cortisol—the body's main stress hormone. Dwellings are meant to be restful spaces—a place you can return to after a busy day at work to relax, allowing cortisol levels (which have typically risen during the working day) to gradually decline. In a cluttered space, cortisol stays risen. This is problematic because in some cases elevated cortisol levels might interfere with learning and memory, weight, blood pressure, and cholesterol levels.

Messy homes also tend to be full of unfinished projects—a shelf that needs putting up or papers that need organizing. The same US study found that living among unfinished projects can lead to feelings of depression and fatigue for those surrounded by stressful reminders of things still to do.

If you compare this to time spent in clutter-free spaces, the reported differences to well-being are huge. Research shows those who live or work in minimalist, clean-lined designs sleep better, feel more organized and in control, and are revitalized after time spent at home. Interestingly, it's estimated 28 percent of employers are less likely to promote someone with a messy workspace.

Happy objects

A largely tidy space, however, will only be fulfilling if it's decorated with objects that make you happy—there's a difference between clutter-free and empty. If you love your home because you have nice artwork, elegant furniture, or family photos on the wall, you're likely to feel more content with life than if you spend time in a space that doesn't make you happy, regardless of any other external factors. You're also more likely to be sociable, inviting others round to share in a space you love. It's sometimes good, therefore, to splash out on that beautiful painting or a new rug if it means you get a rush of joy every time you look at it.

It's also important to choose your color scheme wisely. A splash of paint can make all the difference to the look and feel of a room, but colors can have some surprising consequences on your mood. In fact, color theorists have long spoken of the power that color has in transforming people's way of thinking, which is why study participants state unequivocally that the exact same food tastes far worse when dyed a different color, despite the fact the taste remains unchanged.

A number of studies have found that walls painted red encourage workers to be more productive initially, but over time become more tired and anxious. For example, research by Kwallek and Lewis found that while subjects working in a red office compared to a white one made fewer errors at the start of the experiment, over time the walls became more distracting. This is because the color red has been shown to raise blood pressure, as well as speed respiration and heart rate. It makes people excited and stimulates action, but after prolonged exposure this can have an exhausting reaction for the body. At home, therefore, red is usually considered too stimulating for bedrooms.

In other research, predominantly gray, dull offices were associated with lower levels of enthusiasm, creativity, and productivity. The same goes for gray on the outside—people tend to feel less inspired when surrounded by gray brickwork: so much so that it can lower social aspirations and impede success.

Blue, green, and white, on the other hand, were found to have positive responses from participants. Walls painted with such colors had a significant impact on workers' motivation, productivity, happiness, and inspiration. Blue is said to bring down blood pressure, and slow respiration and heart rate. Green is considered the most restful color for the eye, while white represents youth and cleanliness, and creates a cool, refreshing feeling.

Better by design

Colors can only go so far in influencing the way we feel. More important, perhaps, is the overall design of a room. American biotechnology company Genzyme Corporation created a new corporate headquarters that used natural light, a clear glass exterior, sunlight-reflecting chandeliers, indoor gardens, water features, and windows. Some 18 months after the building opened, 88 percent of workers said the new design had improved their sense of well-being. In part, this is because natural light and access to nature in design does wonders for mental health. Many studies show how workers who have a window with an attractive aspect recover from low-level stress at a much quicker rate than those who have no window. One by Rachel Kaplan found job satisfaction was greater when employees had a view of some natural elements. It was also discovered that the longer participants spent looking out of the window at nature, the more rapidly their heart rate tended to decrease. Again, in studies of call centers, workers who could see the outdoors completed tasks six to seven percent more efficiently than those who couldn't, which generated annual savings of over $2,000 per employee.

The introduction of green plants into a workplace can also make a big difference. Researchers from the University of Cardiff, UK, discovered that workers who introduced natural greenery to their office saw a 15 percent rise in both productivity and creativity over a three-month period, in comparison to those working with no greenery or natural elements within their immediate environment.

Ultimately, the environments in which you spend a lot of time make a big difference to the way you think and feel. Color schemes, how tidy a space is, and how it's designed, all go a long way in determining how beautiful it feels, and therefore how much it improves, or impedes, well-being.

It's easy to live day-to-day, neglecting a messy bookshelf or putting off a redecoration, but in doing so you are missing out on the power a beautiful environment has on your happiness, and most importantly your health.

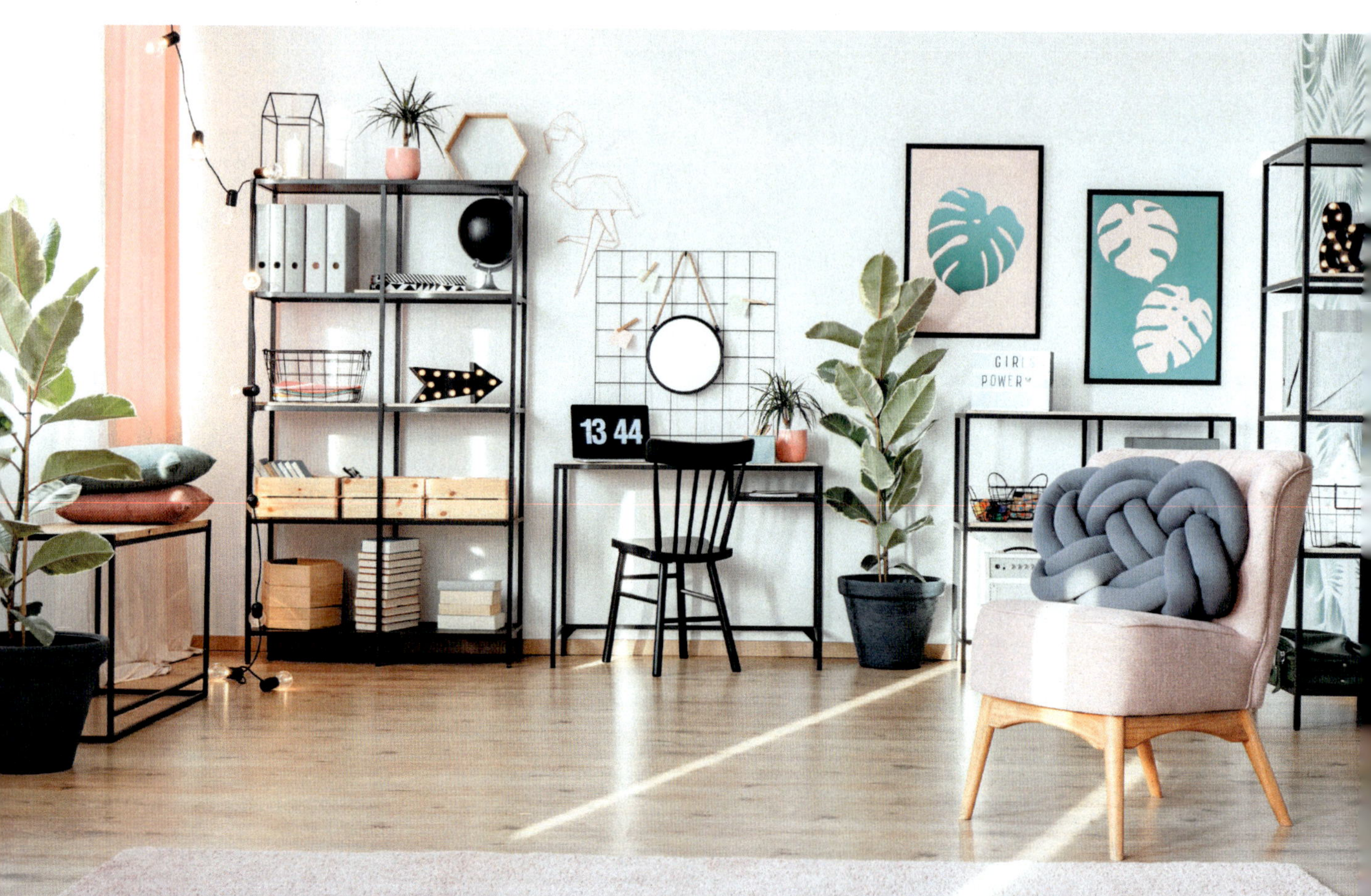

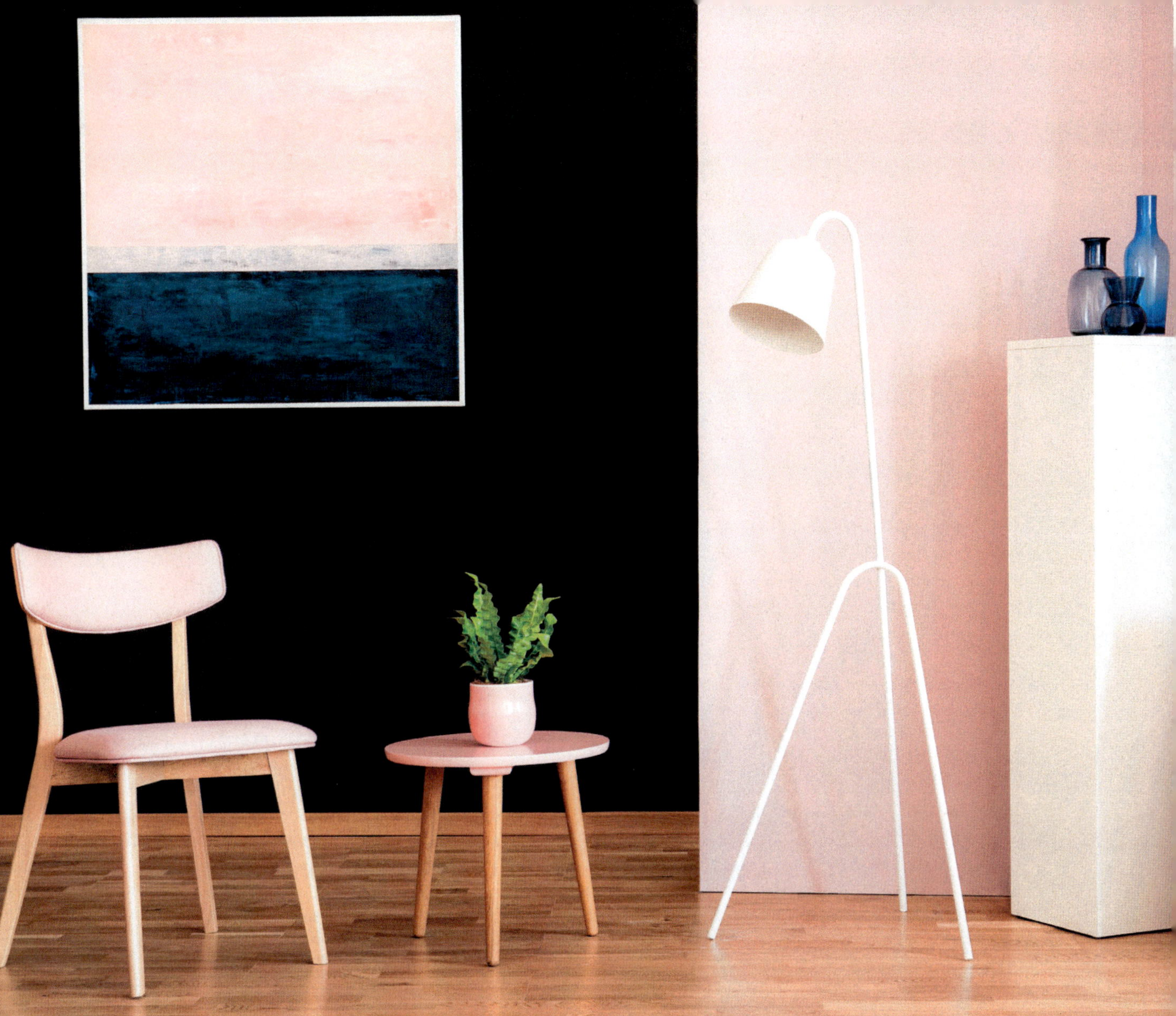

FIVE WAYS TO CULTIVATE BEAUTY AND IMPROVE WELL-BEING

- Put aside time to reorganize your home or office. Start small, with a bookshelf or a messy desk. Properly consider whether you really need to keep that old lamp or stack of dusty magazines. Not only will tidying and decluttering make your space look more attractive, it will also become a place where you can really relax.

- Don't feel guilty about splashing out on making your house look nice. You don't need to spend a fortune—there are plenty of cheap design shops—but a pretty lampshade, nice painting, or colorful rug can go a long way when it comes to improving how beautiful a room looks, and how you feel when you spend time in it.

- Think carefully about your color scheme, as the hues you choose can influence your mood. Neutral colors typically work better in the bedroom as they're more relaxing, while bolder colors suit communal areas. Repainting a feature wall can make a huge difference to the overall look of a room, and it's often a cheap way to feel like you've undergone a bigger redecoration.

- Buy some living green plants for decoration. Not only can they promote productivity and creativity, but houseplants are also good for purifying the air in a room. They add a splash of calming color, too.

- Make the most of your natural light. Consider moving furniture so you sit, work, or sleep closer to a window. If your room doesn't benefit from much natural light, think about opting for a color scheme centered around lighter hues or try hanging some mirrors on the wall—both options can make a space feel lighter, and leave you feeling brighter as well.

Legends of the fall

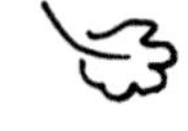

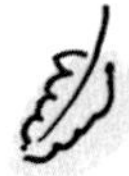

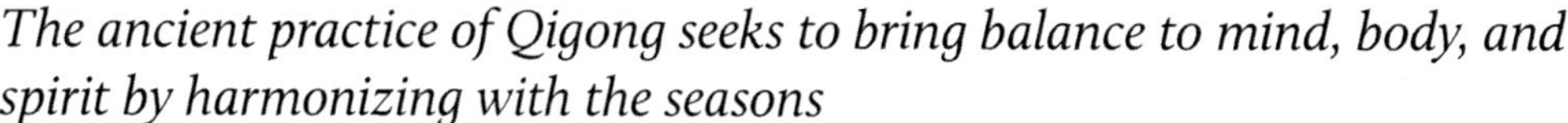

The ancient practice of Qigong seeks to bring balance to mind, body, and spirit by harmonizing with the seasons

The fall equinox is a time of balance. The sun enters Libra as opposing forces of light and dark teeter on a knife edge, before the world slowly begins its descent into longer nights and shorter days. Many give thanks and celebrate the bountiful year, and as the buzz of the turning of seasons tingles the senses, it's almost as if one's own body is ready for hibernation—which, according to Traditional Chinese Medicine (TCM), it is.

Many TCM practitioners believe ignoring this natural instinct to slow down during the fall is a surefire way to wind up with a winter deficit in mind, body, and spirit. The key to good health, happiness, and overall well-being, at any time of year, is finding harmony with the seasons and cycles of life and ensuring internal peace through balance. And the key to the fall season is slowing your pace.

Author and TCM practitioner Christopher Handbury first discovered the Chinese medicine system when his mother, a nurse, introduced him to acupuncture to treat his own chronic migraines—successfully. That was 34 years ago. It was then that his passion for TCM was born and he's now been teaching and practicing for more than 15 years. "TCM is based on the theory that the activity of the body and mind move in specific pathways or vessels," he explains. "They are often described as oceans, rivers, and streams. These pathways carry blood, fluids, and nerve messages to maintain the functions of the organs, tissues, muscles, and bones. When the system is functioning efficiently, we have good health, less illness, and feel a sense of well-being.

"Much like the rivers and streams in life, if they become restricted or blocked the flow can become weak, overbearing, and reduced, creating imbalance. Circulation is affected and the messages do not move freely. When this happens we can feel pain in the physical body and the mind can present emotions that help us to take action and restore the imbalance. It's a natural process, yet one that often feels uncomfortable."

So, what exactly needs to be kept in balance? It's as simple, and as complex, as making sure the combination of the physical body, the spirit, and the emotional mind is working as best as it can. When these three aspects of the self are equally nurtured, with issues arising in any one area being addressed, released, or healed when necessary, this results in a happy and healthy life.

Have you ever felt overwhelmed emotionally and found it left you physically weak and drained? This is an example of one aspect taking over and imbalance arising. When this occurs it must be addressed, or ailments (whether physical, spiritual, or emotional) can follow. According to TCM, there are many ways to treat these imbalances—from acupuncture to herbal treatment.

There is another approach called Qigong, which is a system that combines movement, breath work, self-massage, diet, and harmonizing the seasons and cycles of life. "Qigong is the practice and study of regulating the body and mind through specific methods like active movements, static postures, and breath work," explains Christopher. "In all areas of TCM, including Qigong, each season relates to a specific organ system, body part, and its elemental quality. Within each season certain organs are more vulnerable to the changes in weather, emotions, and climate and Qigong movements are adapted to help with this."

The winding down of the world during the fall is thought to be reflected within the human body. It is considered by many to be a time to take stock of all that you have achieved, and all you hope to achieve in the New Year once you reawaken. It also represents a period of time to be thankful for all that has served and benefitted you in the current year, as well as providing an opportunity to release anything that has not.

The lungs are the organ connected to fall, believed to be the commanders of Wei Qi (protective energy) and the interface between your external and internal worlds. Focusing on building up this energy will help to protect you from winter illness and boost your ability to resist absorbing negativity and imbalance from others around you.

The lungs are also thought of as the physical place where grief, loss, and deep sadness is stored. Using the movement and breath work of Qigong to let go at this time can help you to exhale all that is burdening you and inhale new energy to help rebalance and restore. Doing this in preparation for the cold months ahead can enable the body to journey on with the resilience required to thrive. "Using Qigong in harmony with the season, it is possible to create a strong, resilient, and efficient body and mind that allows us to grow spiritually and discover our true self that so often becomes lost along the way," says Christopher.

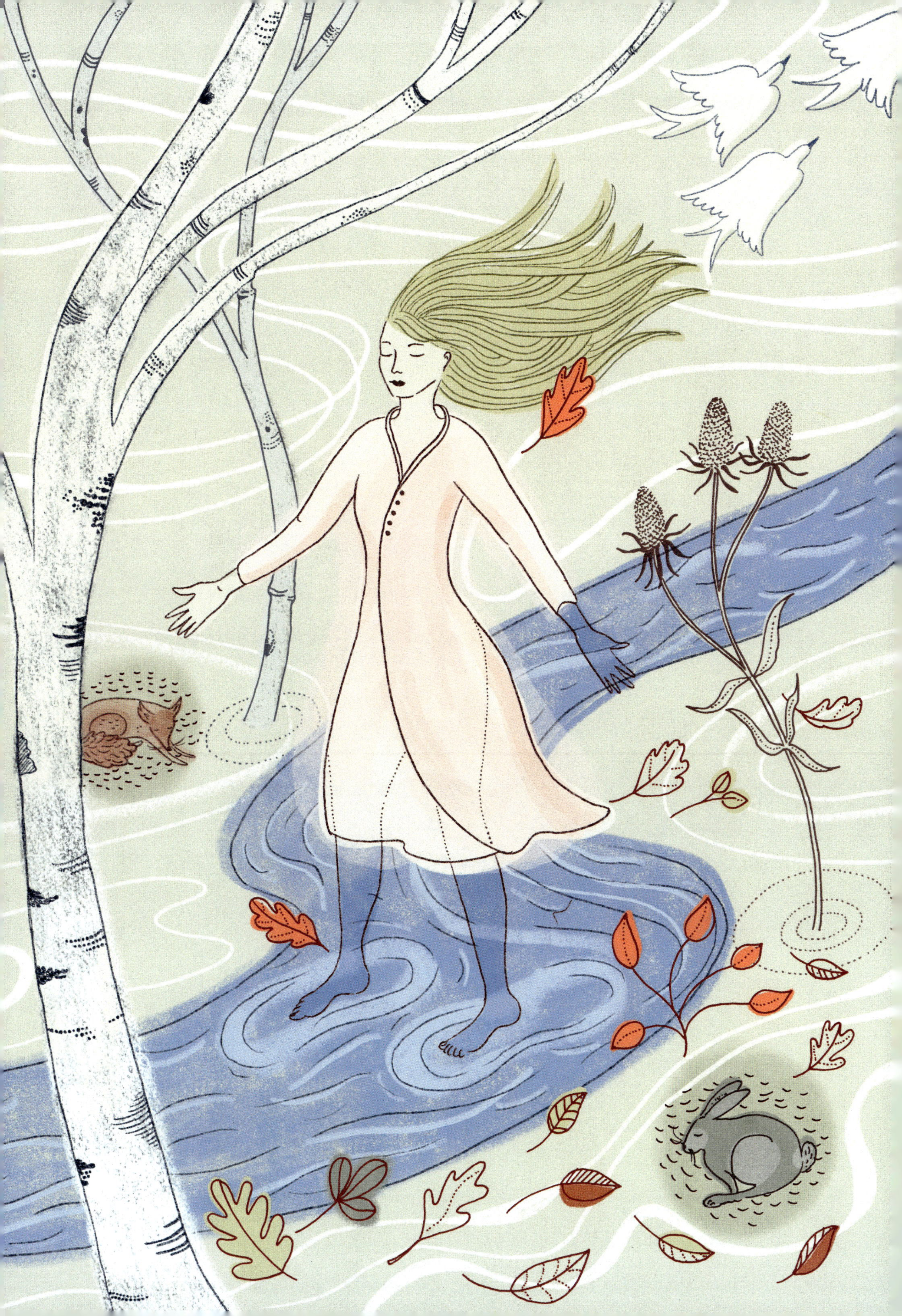

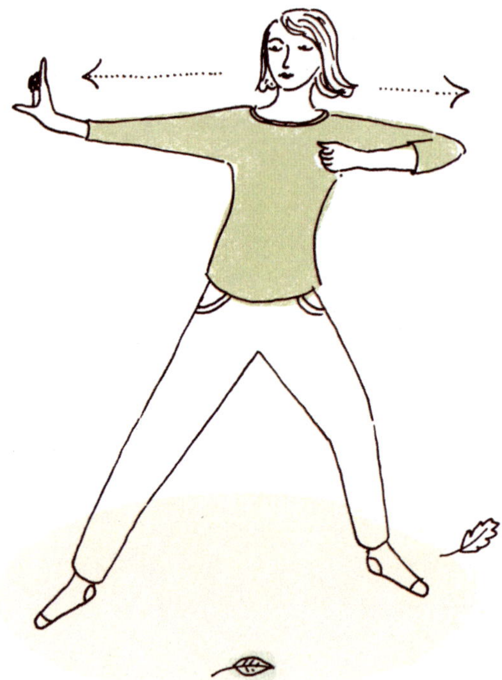

THREE QIGONG MOVEMENTS FOR THE FALL

As with all physical activities, do not attempt any of these movements if you have an injury or medical condition that may be aggravated. If in doubt, always talk to your primary care physician first.

THE INVISIBLE BALL

Use this exercise to strengthen the lung cavity and release the shoulders

- Stand or sit comfortably.
- Hold the arms out in front of the chest as though holding a large ball against your chest.
- Take a relaxed breath and imagine the ball expanding as you separate the arms to the sides.
- When your breath has finished, bring the hands back to the start position while breathing in.

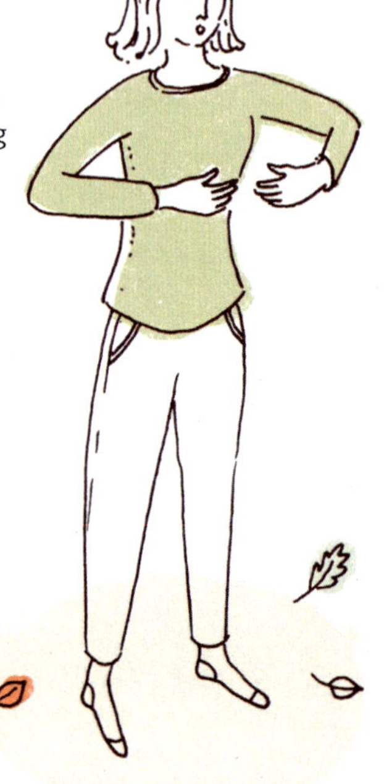

ARCHER DRAWS HIS BOW

This movement helps to strengthen the lungs, stimulate the energy vessels, and exercise the shoulders. It is part of an eight-movement Qigong system that dates back many centuries

- Stand out to the side in a wider-than-shoulder-width stance. Cross the hands in front of your chest with right hand in front, palms facing chest. Sink the weight into the feet and lower the body slightly.
- Loosely clench the left hand as if grasping the string of a bow. At the same time the right hand forms a pointing shape with the thumb out, and the index finger straight upward.
- Raise up the left elbow and pull back as if drawing a bow. Simultaneously move the right arm out to the right until it is fully extended but not locked.
- Now gather the right hand in an arc at shoulder height and return it to the chest. Relax the left hand back toward the body sinking the elbow to rest in front of the chest. You are now back at the beginning. The left hand should be in front of the right.
- Grasp the bow with the right hand and turn the left hand into a pointed hand . . . continue.
- Repeat four times each side.

CARRYING THE MOON

The third movement is said to increase vitality. It's also good for the spine, which is stretched and flexed

- Stand in a central posture with feet hip-width apart.
- Place hands together in front of the abdomen as if holding a balloon.
- Carefully, while hinging at the hips, slowly lower the balloon to the floor until you feel a change in the tissue at the back of the legs. Relax the shoulder to lower the ball a little further.
- When you have reached a comfortable flexion of the waist, begin to raise the arms straight and in an outward arch, maintaining a connection with the rear of the legs.
- When the arms are level with the ears, begin to raise the head and body in line with the arms.
- When you have reached an upward posture, open the hands to form a circle between the thumbs and index fingers as if carrying a ball.
- Separate the hands to the sides, lowering them in an arch, and straighten the body.
- Repeat eight times.

NOURISHING EXTRAS

Immune boost Stimulating the kidneys is a great way to boost the immune system and give your body extra nourishment. To do this—and release your lower back at the same time—place your hands on your lower back and gently massage the area to warm the kidneys after each Qigong movement.

Drive out damp Metal is the fall element in TCM and this is believed to store an excess of damp in the body. When dampness makes its way into the lungs, this can make it much harder to draw new energy in and release the old. Reducing dairy, cold, and greasy foods and enjoying regular saunas is said to help restore equilibrium.

The world on your shoulders Shoulder pain and injuries are common in the fall. Think of this as a reminder that now is the time to try to let go of emotional burdens weighing you down. Pay attention to what your body is doing in response to your emotional landscape—is your chest constricted, protecting your heart? Are you unconsciously reducing your ability to fully breathe, which is resulting in tension in the shoulders? Try to be present at all times and make the choice to willingly let go.

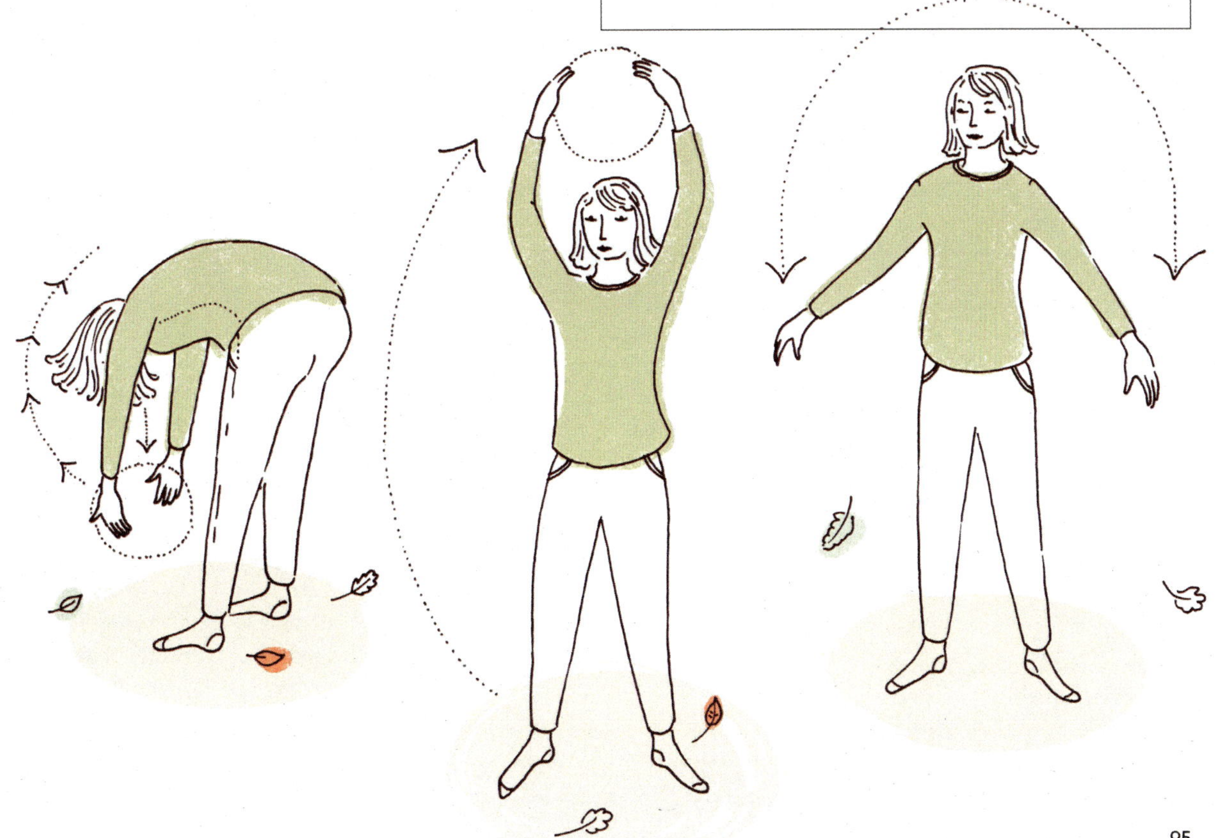

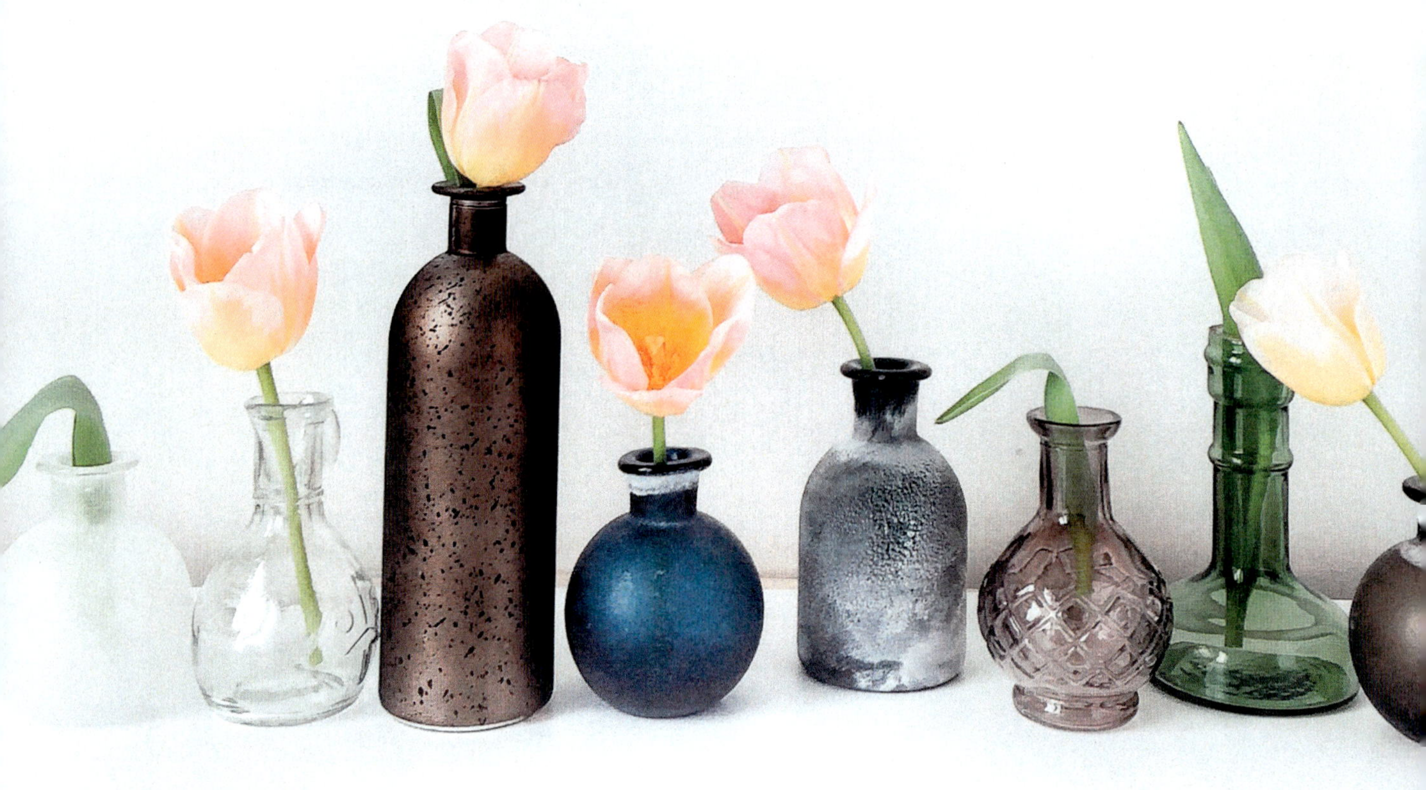

Note to self

Quotes and affirmations that underline the importance of self-care

Our bodies are our gardens, to the which our wills are gardeners.

William Shakespeare

Knowing how to be solitary is central to the art of loving. When we can be alone, we can be with others without using them as a means of escape.

bell hooks

Be you, love you. All ways, always.

Alexandra Elle

The thing that is really hard, and really amazing, is giving up on being perfect and beginning the work of becoming yourself.

Anna Quindlen

To love oneself is the beginning of a lifelong romance.

Oscar Wilde

Almost everything will work again if you unplug it for a few minutes, including you.

Anne Lamot

Keep good company, read good books, love good things, and cultivate soul and body as faithfully as you can.

Louisa May Alcott

If you have the ability to love, love yourself first.

Charles Bukowski

. . . If you feel "burnout" setting in, if you feel demoralized and exhausted, it is best, for the sake of everyone, to withdraw and restore yourself.

Dalai Lama

Had I not created my whole world, I would certainly have died in other people's.

Anaïs Nin

As you grow older, you will discover that you have two hands, one for helping yourself, the other for helping others.

Maya Angelou

When you recover or discover something that nourishes your soul and brings joy, care enough about yourself to make room for it in your life.

Jean Shinoda Bolen

A person learns how to love himself through the simple acts of loving and being loved by someone else.

Haruki Murakami

Made in the USA
Columbia, SC
09 August 2023